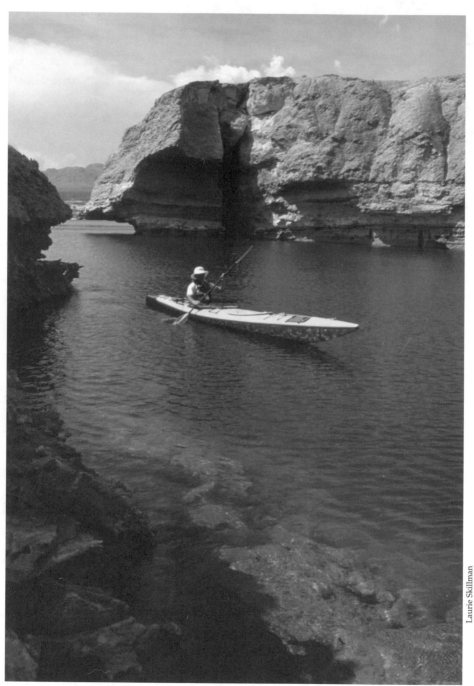

Lake Mead near Bonnelli Bay

Adventure Kayaking

Inland Waters of the Western United States

Includes selected areas in
California, Arizona, Oregon, Nevada
Utah, and Washington

Don Skillman

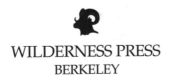

WILDERNESS PRESS
BERKELEY

Copyright © 2000 Don Skillman
FIRST EDITION September 2000

Photos © 2000 Don Skillman, except as noted
Book design by Margaret Copeland—Terragraphics
Maps by the author
Cover photos © 2000 Don Skillman
Cover design by Larry B. Van Dyke

Library of Congress Card Number 00-033555
ISBN 0-89997-250-0

Manufactured in the United States of America
Published by: **Wilderness Press**
             1200 5th Street
             Berkeley, CA 94710
             (800) 443-7227; FAX (510) 558-1696
             mail@wildernesspress.com
             www.wildernesspress.com

             Contact us for a free catalog

Front cover: Kayak camp on Old Devils Lake, Washington
Back cover: *top:* Great Horned Owl
              bottom: Kayak at Rubicon Point, Lake Tahoe, California

♻ Printed on recycled paper, 20% post-consumer waste content

Library of Congress Cataloging-in-Publication Data

Skillman, Don.
     Adventure kayaking : inland waters of the western United States : includes selected
areas in California, Arizona, Oregon, Nevada, Utah, and Washington / Don Skillman.—
1st ed.
        p. cm.
     Includes index.
     ISBN 0-89997-250-0 (alk. paper)
     1. Sea kayaking—West (U.S.)—Guidebooks. 2. Kayak touring—West (U.S.) 3. West
(U.S.)—Guidebooks. I. Title.
GV776.W3 S45 2000
917.904'34—dc21
                                                    00-033555

Table of Contents

Acknowledgments

This book would not exist were it not for my wife Laurie. Her enthusiasm never faltered while traveling the thousands of highway miles necessary to make all the trips in this book. Her willingness as the other paddler in our double kayak made the water miles slip by. She appreciates nature, and brings out the wonder in all things natural. She is an accomplished photographer who sees beauty in nature and captures it as art. Her help in keeping me on track with this book has been invaluable. You the reader will benefit from her contribution to these pages. I treasure her love, companionship, and support.

Thanks to Mike Jones at Wilderness Press, whose quick grasp of concept launched this book. Thanks also to Paul Backhurst, Editor, who lines out the superfluous and massages my sentence structure to within reasonable limits. His help has been invaluable.

Last but not least, a word of appreciation to all of the rangers, recreation specialists, and others at the various state, federal, and tribal agencies who supplied information about waters and regulations. These people helped me just as they stand ready to help you, the kayaker.

Trip Locations

The trip location numbers on this map correspond to the chapter numbers.

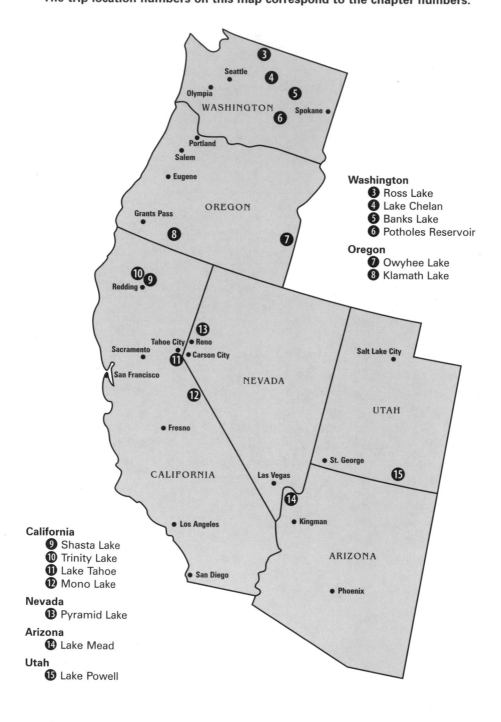

Washington
- **3** Ross Lake
- **4** Lake Chelan
- **5** Banks Lake
- **6** Potholes Reservoir

Oregon
- **7** Owyhee Lake
- **8** Klamath Lake

California
- **9** Shasta Lake
- **10** Trinity Lake
- **11** Lake Tahoe
- **12** Mono Lake

Nevada
- **13** Pyramid Lake

Arizona
- **14** Lake Mead

Utah
- **15** Lake Powell

Introduction

Imagine paddling on large, calm bodies of water that are free of ocean swells and surf. These are the inland lakes and impoundments, waters where thrilling scenery enhances the pure pleasure of cruising in your sea kayak. Open water is what these boats were designed for. Experience a variety of environments and boost your enjoyment level; follow the call of your sleek-lined craft to travel, to explore. Many of these lakes are so big you can kayak for days along the shore. Each lake has a unique personality and setting, which every kayaker can enjoy whether or not she or he is an expert. There are no surf landings, no need to be accomplished at bracing.

This book describes 13 adventure trips for the kayaker on large, inland waters in California, Oregon, Washington, Arizona, Utah, and Nevada. All lakes selected are of sufficient size to facilitate overnight camping from your kayak, an experience that is more than just staying out overnight. The routes offer a real feeling of adventure for you to savor, unique to every lake. Each trip provides the greatest seclusion and wilderness experience possible for the area.

Besides the enjoyable, flat-water paddling which inland waters provide, you will usually be in fresh water. Some inland lakes are salty; Mono Lake for instance, featured in Chapter 12, is far greater in dissolved salts and minerals than is sea water. To a lesser degree, so is Pyramid Lake, in Nevada, described in Chapter 13. Generally speaking, though, inland kayaking is fresh-water paddling. Some of the trips featured in this book are on lakes which occupy a subalpine setting, backed by snowcapped peaks, even in the summer. Lush forests cover the shorelines of other lakes in the middle elevations. Still others are in the semiarid Great Basin, the high desert, or the dry Southwest, their sparkling blue water contrasting sharply with the varicolored rock formations found in interesting desert locales.

There are adventurous kayak-camping trips within an easy day's drive for most kayakers. When exciting alternate trips are possible in the destination area, they are noted. The interesting historical, geological, or natural history features of each trip area are detailed. Included here are all of the contacts you will need to secure up-to-date information on conditions at each trip destination. Permits, fees, and reservations are discussed, so you can take care of these items early in your trip planning. Conditions at each season of the year are described, so you can take your trip when local conditions best suit your schedule. Campgrounds near the launch areas are noted. Driving directions are included to make your trip easy.

The trips detailed here offer routes that can be easily paddled in two days, with a single overnight camp ashore. Some of the routes can be traversed in a single day by strong paddlers. In the case of the larger lakes, especially Lakes Mead and Powell, routes can be extended to a week or more, with trips of hundreds of miles possible. I have paddled all of the trip routes described in this book, and some of the alternate or additional trips. When an alternate or additional trip is suggested which I haven't paddled, this fact will be noted.

If more tranquil water conditions are one factor differentiating inland-water kayaking from coastal paddling, the great variety of environments is the other. The Alaska-like appearance of Washington's Ross Lake contrasts greatly with the desert setting of Potholes Reservoir, also in Washington. Mono Lake, in California, presents an aura vastly different from that on Trinity Lake, in the same state. Lake Powell, with its red-rock cliffs and slick-rock formations, offers yet another uniqueness. Coastal estuaries, and their inland systems, as well as impoundments along the Columbia and Colorado rivers, are not included in this book. Exceptions are Lakes Mead and Powell. While all of these waters are considered inland and certainly meet the size requirements, their similar classifications make them ripe subjects of future books on kayaking west-coast estuaries and river impoundments. Pick a lake or reservoir, select a season, and schedule the date. Read about the area, and procure your maps. You will be visiting the premier inland waters of the Far West. Let the paddling begin.

PART I.

PLANNING & PREPARATION

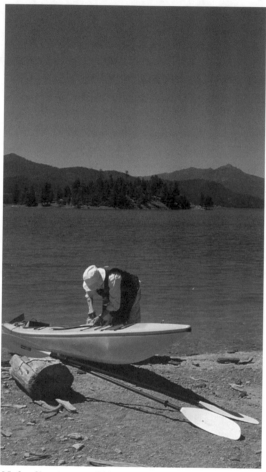

Unloading gear on Trinity Lake shore near Irish Isles

Chapter 1

Planning Your Trip

The purpose of recreational kayaking is enjoyment. Careful planning will ensure that your trip goes smoothly, and that you will see the places and things that are important to you. By planning at home with a chart in hand, you can spot interesting coves you want to explore, and make sure you allow time to do so. With a checklist in hand beforehand, you won't arrive for your trip and find you've left essential equipment at home. Planning will clarify your trip objectives ahead of time, and make it easy for you to reach them.

How to use this book

This book will help you in two ways. It will suggest the premier trips that you've dreamed of, and it will provide all the information you require to take that trip. You need only secure an accurate map for navigation and any necessary permits.

Experience. You don't have to be an experienced kayaker to enjoy the adventure routes in this book. One difference on inland waters compared to kayaking at sea is that conditions are usually more forgiving. You can gain knowledge by reading the books suggested in the bibliography, and considering basic skill lessons offered by kayak shops. Inland, you can paddle, enjoy, and learn, all at the same time. Should conditions deteriorate, you can usually land within a short time.

Ratings. The ratings of each trip in this book are at best only an anticipation of the difficulties that are likely to be encountered. Every trip in this book could be rated "Easy" if water and wind conditions during the trip remained ideal. Should winds start to blow during certain open-water crossings, or while paddling on certain stretches parallel to the wind direction, wave conditions could occur that are above the comfort level of some beginners. This possibility is indicated in the *Hazards* section, and by a rating of "Moderate" rather than, or in addition to, "Easy." The distances covered are well within the capabilities of nearly all beginning paddlers. If you happen to be paddling against the wind, even a slight breeze will mean you must spend more effort over a longer time to travel the same distance. Allow enough time so you won't have to turn your adventure into a marathon.

Time available. To plan your trip, you first need to establish how much time you have available. At the least, you will need sufficient time to travel to the lake you select, paddle the trip route at the pace which is best suited to you, and travel back to your home. To make the trip more enjoyable, allow an extra day or two to either explore other options in the area, or wait out more favorable weather conditions sometime during your trip. Paddling is much safer, and more gratifying, when *you* decide when to paddle instead of being pressured by an inflexible schedule.

Occasionally your available time will dictate considering a nearby destination, even though the season of the year may not be optimal for paddling there. Only you can make judgment calls of that sort. If you are considering an off-season trip, a call to the ranger station, campground, or other area facility can give you information on what the weather is like. Seasonal variations are very common, so don't count out a beautiful mountain lake just because it's late fall; the area just might be experiencing a fantastic period of unseasonably warm and sunny days.

Season. If time is the first consideration, the season of the year is an important second. You probably wouldn't try to paddle Ross Lake in the dead of winter; you couldn't get there. And unless you are a fan of hot weather, postpone your Lake Mead trip until the heat of summer has moderated. The *When To Go* sections in each chapter outline the general conditions that can be expected in an area for that season of the year, giving you enough information to decide when to make your trip.

Water levels. Some of the trips in this book are on reservoirs. A few of these reservoirs have water levels that can vary widely depending upon season, precipitation, the multi-season trend of drought or above-average precipitation, and even upon factors unrelated to weather patterns. Exactly when you paddle on reservoirs with wide fluctuations in water levels will affect your trip to some degree. When a reservoir is full, it is said to be at "full pool," in other words, the water level is as high as it gets. Being at full pool means various things to the paddler. First of all, the lake level will be up to the undisturbed shoreline, be it wooded or bare rock. When the lake is full, water extends back into all the coves and inlets, enhancing aesthetics. Now, availability of camping areas depends upon the configuration of the shoreline above the high watermark.

While the visual impact of a bare shoreline, exposed when the water level is down 30 feet or so, is probably not your first choice, that condition doesn't mean the end of your trip plans. Some inlets and arms may be shortened considerably at very low water levels, but there is plenty of water left upon which to kayak. And there's one bonus of lower water levels: campsites are virtually everywhere. This is because many knolls, ridges, and alluvial beaches, which were underwater at full pool, are now exposed, free of vegetation, and just waiting for you to camp there. You can go ashore almost anywhere. When you inquire of administrative agencies about a specific lake or reservoir, always ask about the water level to get an idea of what to expect. If there are severe water-level conditions that would make rescheduling your trip on a particular reservoir advisable, you will know about them.

Maps. You will need to secure the necessary maps for your trip before you leave. If maps such as USGS quadrangles are not available near you, they must be ordered by mail, a process that can require a week or two. Once you have the map or chart of your selected trip in hand, the process of planning your trip is greatly enhanced. Your maps will show much more detail than those in this book, which are for orientation only and not intended for navigation. You can order USGS maps from the government at the least cost, but delivery may be slow. If you are in a hurry, there are private companies that can ship most USGS maps to you the same day you order for a higher price. These companies are listed in Appendix 1.

Transportation. You will probably be driving an automobile to the trip location, and carrying along your kayak. Most state road maps will be sufficiently detailed that you'll have no trouble driving to the location, using the directions given in each chapter. All paddling routes are round trips, designed to return you to the starting point.

Your kayak

Most kayaks fall into several categories, depending upon the purpose for which they were designed. White-water kayaks are very low-volume boats designed for maneuverability in river currents. They are not supposed to keep the paddler dry or carry any gear, and are highly specialized. Play boats designed for general purposes include sit-upon kayaks among other designs, which are not suitable for serious cruising uses. Sea kayaks, on the other hand, are generally higher-volume boats designed for cruising and fitted with rudders. Their cockpits are designed with coamings that form seals with the paddlers' spray skirts. Sea kayaks are the type most suitable for the trips described in this book.

Choose a sea kayak that provides: sufficient volume to carry you and your touring gear and supplies; sufficient length to facilitate easy tracking and the best speed; and, the lowest profile to reduce windage (consistent with the other requirements). The type of material from which a kayak is made is not of major importance, provided it is of high quality. Some materials have inherent manufacturing limitations that preclude their use in certain designs. Fiberglass is a common material, especially for larger boats, while polyethylene is less expensive and has greater resistance to hull scratching. With quality components and workmanship, the design itself is more important than the type of material used.

Your paddle. On a par with the performance of your kayak is the performance of your paddle. Consider that you will be making up to 30 individual strokes with a paddle blade each minute; you will dip a blade as many as 1,800 times each hour. Since you hold the paddle in your arms, it goes without saying that its light weight is an important feature. Also, the weight of the blades and shaft should be balanced in a way that makes the paddle feel good when you use it. A poor paddle will feel stiff and clublike. While blade shape is an individual choice, good design will allow you to dip and recover the paddle without unduly disturbing the water, yet provide sufficient surface to transfer the energy of your stroke efficiently. Be sure to use a paddle long enough that you aren't hitting the side of your boat during your normal stroke.

Paddles are either one piece, or two piece. They may be feathered with the blades at an offset angle to one another, or straight with the blade surfaces parallel. Being able to use the paddle either feathered or straight is a feature of some two-piece models. Such paddles also may be easier to pack, since they can be taken apart to reduce their length. Most good paddles are somewhat expensive, but are worth the cost.

It is not the purpose of this book to be a how-to guide on kayaking in general, or even kayak touring. Many excellent volumes have been written that are specific to kayaking techniques and navigation. Some of these are listed in the bibliography.

Renting kayaks

Since few rental possibilities exist at the trip sites in this book, plan to rent a boat where you live and take it with you. Because demand may make rental boats scarce during peak times of the year, plan to make your reservations well ahead. Let the rental company know what type of trip you are taking, and consider their experience if they recommend a specific type or brand of boat.

Most rental paddles are good, but some are not. If you are fairly certain you will continue in the sport of kayaking but will be renting boats for a while, it may be smart to buy your own paddle. You won't have to buy it later, when you procure your own boat. The same advice holds true for your life vest, and even your spray skirt provided a standard size is used.

Boating laws

Muscle-powered craft are regulated less than any other type of boat. This does not mean that we should be irresponsible in their use, however. Most states have adopted laws that regulate boat use on inland waters, and these laws change from time to time. The U.S. Coast Guard requirements parallel the state laws, but may have additional requirements. Laws set forth the equipment each boat must carry. Aside from a universal requirement that there must be life jackets aboard for each passenger, sound-making devices and a light source capable of being seen at night may be required. To make sure you are in compliance, inquire at your trip destination before you paddle or make inquiries of the state involved. Most have comprehensive booklets detailing their regulations. Contact information is provided in Appendix 1.

Fishing

Some paddle-boat adventurers like to fish on trips, while others do not. In some very remote environments, fishing is a problem because fish odor can mean a visit by a bear. The trips in this book are in areas where bear problems are unlikely, if reasonable precautions are taken. But if you do fish, and your trip is on a lake surrounded by forest, you may want to take extra precautions to avoid having a strong fish smell on your kayak, gear, or on you. Inquire locally to determine if bears are present and, if so, how persistent they are. It is your responsibility not to allow any bear to secure food from any human, not even one time. Be sure to follow the local agency recommendations for environmentally friendly disposal of fish innards.

To fish in any of the waters described in this book, you will need a fishing license issued by the state in which the water is located. Pyramid Lake in Nevada, described in Chapter 13, is the sole exception; this lake is owned by the Pyramid Lake Paiute Tribe, which issues their own permits. If you fish there, make sure you get a permit first.

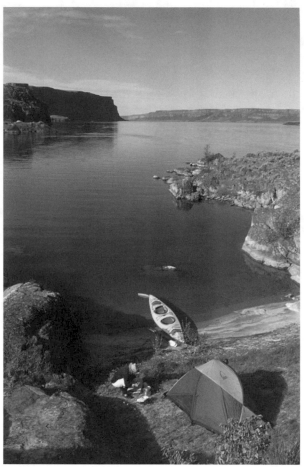

Cozy camp at north end of Old Devils Lake offers a fine gravel beach and views of Steamboat Rock

Chapter 2

Kayak Camping

Campsites

The ability to recognize or find campsites is perhaps the most important skill ensuring enjoyable kayaking. You will probably spend more time in camp than you do on the water. This is especially true if your trip lasts for several days and several different camps are involved. From your living room, it is easy to imagine a sandy beach with kayaks drawn up, your tent pitched on a grassy spot beside a shade tree watered by a tinkling brook, all with a west-facing view that features a magnificent sunset reflecting in the glassy waters of the cove. Such camps exist, but often there is an ingredient or two lacking. In extreme circumstances, *all* features of the campsite are lacking except a spot that allows you to land alive. The vast majority—if not all—of your camps will be somewhere in between. Knowing how to search for, and find, the best available campsites will add pleasure to your paddle expeditions.

Two essential elements of a campsite

The first essential element of a campsite is somewhere to land your boat. This should be a place where you can get off the water safely, and unload your gear. The second most important element is a fairly level spot large enough for your tent, with a somewhat smooth surface. If necessary, you can prop your portable stove on a round boulder, sit upon another, and manage your camp routine without a level or open area. But few will want to pitch their tent and sleep that way. So a place to erect your tent is essential.

A minimal campsite, then, is a place where you can land and put up your tent. If there is a level place to cook and lounge, so much the better. If this hypothetical site also has a view, you will enjoy your stay more. If you don't have to carry your gear a long way, it is even better. Being able to see your boat from the campsite is also nice. In areas where good campsites are not plentiful or just plain do not exist, you may have to accept less favorable conditions. Sometimes the only possible site dictates that you carry your gear a hundred yards or so, uphill. Such a place wouldn't qualify as a *good* campsite, but you'll use it if it is the *only* campsite. You're in business if you find a good place to land and a suitable place nearby to pitch your tent. Other amenities, such as space, shade, access to running water, view—the elements that make a perfect site—are not always there when you want them.

Often you can find a good place to land your boat, but the shore is too steep—or brushy or rocky—to pitch your tent. If you don't want to paddle to the next possible site, search inland a reasonable distance for a suitable spot for your tent. Good bets are small knolls, where a gentle, convex surface usually means that there is a flat place at the top for your tent. Other good places to look are on ridges, or points projecting out into the water. Such landforms, which break up the side slope, and provide convex surfaces that blend into it gradually, offer small flat areas. When knolls or ridges are apparently covered with vegetation as you view them from water level, on top there will be wider spacing between plants, or open areas, large enough for your tent. In vegetation-covered country, large trees often shade out the understory, leaving a

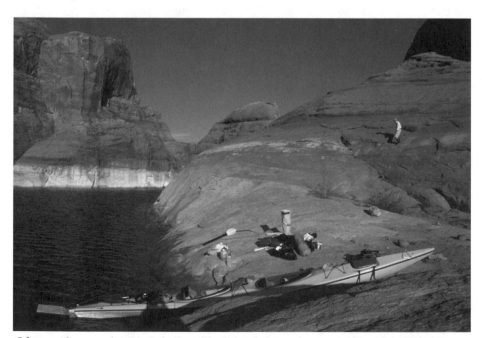

Often sand accumulates in Lake Powell's slickrock depressions, providing tent platforms

brush-free area beneath. If this opening is large enough and acceptably level, you've found a campsite. Most campsites are located in coves and at the heads of bays. This is because water-borne material usually fills in the bottom of inlets to form beaches and gentler slopes, or wave action has concentrated sand or gravel at that spot. The only caveat: if this head-of-the-cove spot is in desert country with the possibility of a flash flood, don't camp there. Camp on suitable high spots to avoid this hazard of desert terrain.

Sometimes you may spot a dream campsite, but there is no place to land your boat. Most landing sites are narrow mud or gravel portions of beach on a manageable slope, with room between rocks to maneuver your boat. Many paddlers have had the experience of exiting their boats among boulders, stepping into water or onto a slippery surface while attempting to hold their craft off the rocks. If the shore is precipitous or there are waves running, such landings are dangerous and should be avoided. But if you can manage the landing and the site is tantalizing enough, the judgment call is yours.

Some highly controlled waterways, such as high-use areas in National Parks, specify which campsites you must use. Your trip must be fully anticipated and planned on such waters, with each night in a specific camp. Only the direst of emergencies will justify deviation from your plan. One advantage of this system is that you will always have a campsite no matter what the competition, and you know in advance where it is. Such controls also concentrate camping impact in specific, limited areas, while allowing minimal structures such as docks, tables, and (most important) toilets. You trade a certain amount of independence, adventure, and solitude for this camp-reservation system.

Sometimes conditions can dictate that you make camp very soon. Illness, fatigue, darkness, storm, or wind can singly, or in concert, make it imperative that you find a place to land. Hopefully this will also be a place where you can camp. One campsite in Southeast Alaska's Inland Passage comes to mind, at the end of a day when we had paddled for hours in deteriorating conditions, along a shore consisting of vertical cliffs descending into tidewater. Darkness was minutes away when we finally found a jumble of talus that looked climbable, and upon which we could land without stoving in our double boat. It wasn't fun wrestling that boat up slippery boulders to safety above the tideline, nor carrying our gear 50 feet up the very steep slide to where—with the addition of some brush and moss—the craggy top of a huge rock served as a tent platform. But it was the best option at the time.

When the weather is excellent, the water calm, and the day early, you can take your time in selecting just the right spot from those possibilities you find. If promising places are few and far between, you can always paddle on until you either find your ideal campsite, or are willing to settle for what is available. Even if paddling a certain number of miles or hours is one of your daily goals, it is best to remain flexible. That "perfect" site might come along an hour before you planned to stop. Take it, unless you know for sure where the next site is located.

Environmental ethics

By just being out on the water in our kayak, we produce an impact. This impact may be only the sight of us by another solitude-seeking kayaker, or it may be the panicked fleeing of a brood of just-hatched mergansers, which weren't seen until the boat drew too close. Whatever it might be, there is an impact that carries with it a clear *responsibility*. Although it would seem our impact while paddling ceases after we pass, it is not really the case. The other paddler still feels our presence, and a panic-stricken duckling may be too stressed to survive. There is always an impact.

If the impact of our paddling seems to disappear after we've passed, it can be the opposite when we camp. Here we leave marks in the mud, flattened grass under the tent, scuffed plants where we squatted while cooking, and upturned rocks which held our tent. While we cannot avoid all impact ashore, there are ways to mitigate that impact. Select campsites that are void of vegetation, if you can find them. Sand and small gravel can withstand the surface disturbance of camping with no lasting damage. If you move rocks or any other material, replace these before you leave. This is especially important when campsites are few and far between, for it is almost certain that others will be using the same site in the future.

Select your tent and other gear in subdued colors, to minimize your visual impact when camping on the shore. Mountaineering tents are often brightly colored so they will stand out, an aid in finding your way back to them. This is not so important in kayak camping, because when you leave, you'll probably take your camp with you; so don't hesitate to use an earth-tone or camouflage tent if one is available. Boat colors are another matter. Manufacturers use bright hull colors as a marketing tool, and the high visibility of such boats is a safety factor on the water, offsetting any negative visual objections. And while you probably also want your paddle jacket and life vest to be highly visible for safety reasons, your gear in camp can be more subdued.

Sanitation. Human excrement should always be carried out, and on many popular rivers that is a requirement. This is accomplished by various systems using plastic bags that can be carried and are odor free. One method in common use involves defecating on a scrap of paper, such as a square cut from a paper bag. When you're finished, pick up the feces in the folded paper, and drop it into a plastic bag, and then tightly close it. Upon return, dispose of the waste in special containers or—if none are provided—into *pit* (not flush) toilets.

If carrying out your feces is not possible, the proven system of using "cat holes" is the next best method. Dig a small hole 4-6" deep, defecate, and replace the earth. Carry out all toilet paper. The location chosen for the hole is far more important than how deep it is. Select the brushiest, least-likely-to-be-visited spot you can find, the farther from camp and water sources the better. We are not talking a few yards here, but hundreds of feet. Even in moist climates, with plenty of soil microbes, complete underground decomposition of feces is a slow process. Do all you can to avoid creating one big outhouse in outdoor areas.

Camping gear

If you backpack, you already have most of the gear for comfortable kayak camping. All that is really required is some form of shelter (tent), sleeping bag, a stove and pot for cooking, and eating utensils. Admittedly, this is an austere list. In reality you will probably take a few more than these five items, but comfortable kayak camping *requires* no more gear than you would take along on a backpack trip. Even better, the same gear will suffice.

Sleeping bags. If you want to specialize your gear for kayaking, the first item to look at is your sleeping bag. Down bags are superior for backpacking because they provide the greatest warmth for the weight. But down gets wet

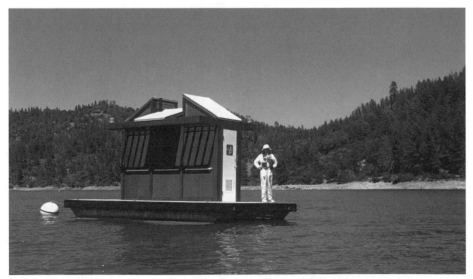

The Forest Service provides floating convenience stations on Shasta Lake

easily, and when wet provides poor insulation. Polyester fillings, while more bulky and less efficient than down, continue to insulate effectively when wet or damp. Therefore, the ideal bags for the water environment of kayaking are those filled with polyester. Use compression straps to reduce the size of a stuffed polyester bag before placing it in a waterproof dry bag.

Tents. You can select tents with those features that are best suited for kayaking. The size, or bulk, of the packed tent is more important than the weight, because while loading your kayak, you are more likely to run out of space before the weight of your gear overloads the boat. Look for tents that are free-standing, because such tents are easiest to pitch if campsite size is limited. Tent size should be no larger than two-person, for the same reason. Choose a tent that is designed to withstand winds, with guyline attachment points, and a fly that does not flap loosely to keep you awake if the wind does blow. A good tent is essential gear. It prevents insect bites while you sleep, and guards against crawly things in your sleeping bag or clothing. More important, it protects you and your gear from precipitation, and shelters you from wind chill.

Stoves. Portable stoves are an absolute necessity. The days when wood-fueled campfires were acceptable in wilderness, desert, undeveloped outdoor areas, or along the shoreline of lakes described in this book, are long gone. The obvious wildfire danger aside, wood fires create long-lasting impact on the sites. They also abort the natural recycling of nutrients since wood is burned and not left to decay. The only justified uses of backcountry wood fires are as signals or heat sources in true life-threatening situations.

Cooking on a small portable stove is much easier than on a wood fire. You don't need a grate or grill, because your stove provides a platform for utensils. Its weight is minimal, even with enough fuel for an extended trip. Though white gas is the preferred fuel, better stoves will burn automotive fuel and even kerosene as well. State-of-the-art stoves allow you to also control heat, from simmer to high flame. Make sure your stove provides a windscreen, since most cooking takes place out in the open. While butane or propane gas-cartridge stoves are easy to light, carrying empty cartridges for later disposal is a considerable disadvantage. Usually such cartridges are not refillable, and only add to landfills.

Sunshades. Since some of the trips described in this book are in warm climates, a word about sunshades may be helpful. Some manufacturers advertise sunshades, often with support structures. Most of these are heavy, bulky, and will not withstand wind. It is better to use a very lightweight, ripstop nylon tarp, in the 2-oz.-per-yard range, and preferably coated with polyurethane so it will shed rain. Make certain there are substantial grommets at the corners, and every 2 feet on the sides. A good size is 8x10 feet.

If there are trees where you camp, pitching the shade is easy, but you probably don't need it. Shades are most helpful out in the open, say in the desert or on a sandy beach. Use your paddle for a pole. Tie one side of the tarp to the end of the blade of a single paddle, or two corners to the blades of two paddles, and guy the paddles down to anchors such as stakes, rocks, driftwood, or bushes. Pull out the opposite side of the tarp, and anchor to the ground in the same manner, or by piling rocks along the edge. You should now have a lean-to sunshade. The methods of anchoring vary according to the site and available materials. Whatever you use for anchors, be sure to put them back where you found them. Leave the site pristine.

Chairs. One of the nice things about kayaks is their ability to carry a generous amount of gear. You have options in taking items that add to your comfort in camp. One item to consider is a canvas backrest, or chair. Some models will work even if you slide out the rigid foam seat and back, making them less bulky. Such supports are ideal when you must spend a lot of time in your tent.

Rain gear. Parkas and raincoats serve well while paddling and on shore. Rain hats with wide brims drip water away from you, and work better than hoods. Paddling jackets, with closures at the neck and wrists, have advantages while paddling and can be used as rain jackets ashore. Rain pants will keep you dry in camp, and can keep you warm if worn while paddling. Breathable rain garments, if they are top quality, cause less condensation and are more comfortable to wear.

Footwear. Everyone has his or her favorite, but for simplicity and utility it's hard to beat knee-high rubber boots. They allow you to embark or land while keeping your feet dry, and are supportive enough to wear in camp. If you contemplate hiking as part of your trip, take separate hiking shoes or boots.

Clothing. For kayaking in warm climates, you can wear cotton clothing. If you get cotton clothes wet, they will cool you through evaporation for a long time. This is the very reason why, if kayaking in colder climates, you should not wear cotton. In this case, use polyester clothing, especially as the first layer. Nylon and other synthetics absorb little moisture, insulate even when wet, and are excellent for layering. Remember that wind penetrates loosely-woven synthetics easily, so use a wind shell, such as your parka and wind pants, to avoid loosing body heat to wind.

Equipment list (May double as packing list)

for Boat
  kayak
  paddle
  extra paddle
  life jacket
  spray skirt
  bilge pump
  paddle float
  rope self-rescue sling or step
  cockpit cover
  boat-repair kit
  dry bags
  bow line
  additional light line
  compass
  charts or maps
  sponge
  water canteen

for Safety
  wet suit or dry suit
  flares
  flashlight
  signal mirror
  weather radio
  barometer/altimeter
  lighter, matches in waterproof container

for Camping
  tent with fly, stakes, wind guys, extra nylon cord
  sunshade
  sleeping bag & pad
  stove
  fuel for stove
  matches and lighter kept with stove
  cooking pot
  bowl
  spoon
  cup
  water filter or treatment tablets
  water bags or containers for 2-day supply

for Personal Use
  prescription medications
  sunglasses, with strap
  first-aid kit
  wilderness medicine guide
  sunscreen (15 or above)
  insect repellent
  personal toiletry items
  camera & film
  mini binoculars
  entertainment items (books, cards)

The above lists contain items that most paddlers will consider as essential. But no two lists will be exactly alike. To decide on including an item, apply this test: Can you get along without it? Or, for safety items: Is deleting this an unacceptable risk? Depending upon your answer, you may decide that the item is an absolute necessity, or else merely a gadget not worth the trouble. But realize that these decisions will vary greatly because of differences in experience and expectations of the people making them.

Food

What food to take on a paddle trip is also a very personal matter. For those who enjoy cooking outdoors, choices will probably include dinners that require some cooking time and effort. Others may opt for packaged, pre-cooked, freeze-dried dinners, which only require boiling water and are ready in minutes. There are environmental ethics to be considered by all, however. Cooked dinners may involve disposal of excess or burned foodstuff, while freeze-dried users always accumulate empty packaging. The only way to avoid negative impact to any inland water is to carry out any excess or burned food, and any packaging. Leave nothing on land or in the water at your campsite.

It takes only a little time and effort to be environmentally responsible. The ideal is no trace, no impact. Strive toward this objective anytime you are in the outdoors. Not only will doing so increase your enjoyment, but the memories of your trip will be more pleasant, knowing that you have done your part to preserve the natural features we love.

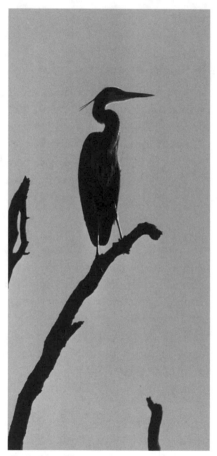

*Great blue heron—classic sentinel of
natural, undisturbed waters*

PART II.

PACIFIC NORTHWEST

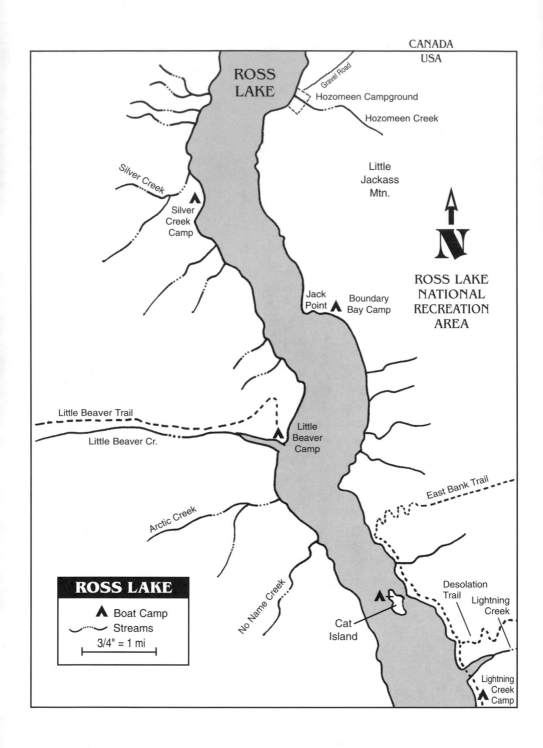

Washington

Chapter 3

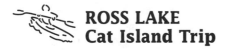

ROSS LAKE
Cat Island Trip

Trip Details	
Distance:	17 miles
Time:	7 hours paddling
Rating:	Easy to Moderate
Maps:	USGS 7.5-min: *Hozomeen Mountain*, *Pumpkin Mountain*, and *Ross Dam*

Summary and Highlights

Ross Lake offers a fantastic, flat-water paddle in a fjordlike wilderness setting. While actually a reservoir, the lake has the aura of true wilderness. Early season runoff causes thundering waterfalls at locations along the shore. Snowfields dot surrounding peaks, adding perpetual glaciers to the views. Precipitous shorelines are timbered with old-growth conifers. The 24-mile-long lake is large enough to distribute usage, which is never high, further enhancing the paddling experience. Shoreline boat camping is by permit only, a Park Service system that controls the number of campers. Vehicle access to the lake is from the north, through Canada. There are 19 boat camps on the lake, and extended paddle trips are possible (see Additional or Alternate Trips later in this chapter).

Boat camping permits, which are issued at Hozomeen at the north end of the lake, and at Marblemount Ranger Station on Highway 20 in Washington, are on a first-come, first-served basis. Day paddling does not require a permit, so you can take day trips if you have to wait your turn for a permit.

Best time to go: Ross Lake is at or near full-pool levels from June to September, depending upon snowpack runoff and hydroelectric demand.

High water levels improve the scenic value, and give easiest access to docks at the improved boat camps. Access to the lake is practical during the summer season only. For the greatest seclusion, and also the best chance to secure a permit, time your trip to avoid weekends and holiday periods.

Hazards: As on any large body of water, sudden wind and the consequent waves are the major safety concern for paddlers. Ross Lake is aligned with the prevailing winds, and open-water stretches of several miles allow sizable wind waves to build up. Traveling along the east shore, where there are more landing sites and more protection, is safest. Paddling early in the day and close to shore are ways to minimize being caught in conditions that are outside your comfort limits. Water temperature in the lake seldom rises above 55°F, so cold water must be considered a hazard. Also, be sure to treat or filter any lake or stream water you intend to drink. Water for cooking needn't be treated if it is boiled for a few minutes.

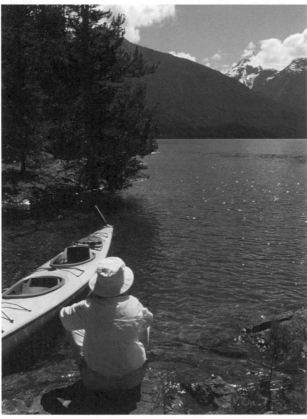

Cat Island's west-shore landing site offers a great view of North Cascade glaciers

Black bears are present at Ross Lake, and occasionally a grizzly bear visits the region. Be sure to camp as odor-free as possible, either bear-bagging your food or using bear-proof storage boxes where provided.

Mosquitoes are most numerous early in the season. These pests are scarce out on the water, but can be bothersome in camp. Take long pants and long-sleeve shirts, as well as repellent.

How to Get There

The only vehicle access to Ross Lake is at Hozomeen, at the north end of the lake just south of the Canada border. Take Trans-Canada Highway 1 in British Columbia from Vancouver east to Hope. At the junction of Old Highway 1 in Hope, go approximately 1 mile west on that route to a signed road that leads left (south) to Silver and Ross lakes. Proceed 39 miles south on this road to Hozomeen. The first several miles are paved; beyond that the road degrades to a gravel surface.

Hozomeen consists of a ranger station and residences, and a lakeside campground with pit toilets, fire rings, tables, and water. There are minimal launching ramps and docking facilities. Hozomeen is located in Ross Lake National Recreation Area, and is administered by the National Park Service. Boat-camping permits can be obtained from rangers here.

The other practical access to Ross Lake is from Highway 20 (the North Cascades Highway), which leads east from Burlington, WA. Take Hwy. 20 to Diablo Dam, just a few miles west of Ross Dam on the Skagit River. Launch at Diablo Dam, or at Colonial Creek, and paddle east 4 miles on Diablo Lake to Ross Dam. With prior notice and a reservation, Ross Lake Resort will portage your kayak and gear around Ross Dam and deposit you on Ross Lake for a small fee. More about Ross Lake Resort can be found under Contacts later in this chapter.

Area Features, Background, and Tips

The northern Cascade Mountains in western Washington are a potpourri of jagged peaks, glaciers, streams, rivers, and waterfalls, separated by U-shaped, glacial-cut canyons now clad in lush conifer forests. The highest peaks in the region are in the subalpine and alpine elevations of 8,000-9,000 feet, jutting well above timberline, which is around 6,000 feet at this latitude. From your kayak on the surface of Ross Lake, you can view perpetual glaciers sculpting the mountain tops.

Cross-country hiking is difficult if not impossible here because of topography and the lush growth of alders, willows, vine maples, and devil's club. A few trails access the backcountry. These are discussed in the Trip Description later below.

Modern exploration of the North Cascades began in 1814 when Alexander Ross passed through while on an expedition to "discover" the area. In 1859 Henry Custer, on a reconnaissance mission for the International Boundary Commission, noted in his journal that "Mountain masses and peaks present strange, fantastic, dauntless, and startling outlines." It is no different today. Access to the area has been improved by construction of one highway and a handful of trails, but that's it. This area of the Northwest is where wolves live and howl, and the occasional grizzly bear spreads awe from the top of the food web.

North Cascades National Park and Ross Lake and Lake Chelan National Recreation Areas were established in 1968. Stephen Mather, first director of the National Park Service, was honored in 1988 when 93% of the total of park and recreation areas here was declared the Stephen Mather Wilderness, adding yet another layer of administrative protection. All three areas comprise a contiguous block of nearly three quarters of a million acres. Bordering lands to the south, east, and west are National Forest. Across the international border to the north lies Skagit Valley Provincial Park. The result is a biological corridor along the crest of the Cascade Mountains from the Columbia River well into Canada. And you can paddle into the heart of it.

A scant handful of explorers and prospectors visited the region in the late 1800s and early 1900s. A little mining was done and then abandoned because transportation was so difficult in such a remote and rugged area. Between 1924 and 1961, Seattle City Light constructed three hydroelectric dams on the Skagit River, all of which are now within the 117,000-acre Ross Lake National Recreation Area. This action effectively cut off salmon runs to the upper Skagit River spawning grounds upstream from the dams. Fishing is fair in Ross Lake for rainbow, eastern brook, and cutthroat trout. Washington game and fish regulations apply. While there are bull trout as well as Dolly Varden in Ross Lake, these species must be released and cannot be taken.

Similar in aura to a Southeast Alaskan fjord, shorelines are generally steep—even precipitous—and carpeted with lush, old-growth conifers. A number of waterfalls plunge into the lake at various locations, heavy in their flows during times of snowmelt. Adjacent peaks nurture glaciers and year-round snowfields. Early season promises more extensive snow-clad areas near, but still above, the lake.

While not a mecca for wildlife in terms of abundance, you may see or hear common loons, ospreys, kingfishers, blue herons, and an occasional bald eagle. There are black bears during the paddling season, and the slight chance of a grizzly's visit. Wolves are present but seldom seen or heard. Mountain goats and deer each stick to their own habitat. Mountain lions are rare, and signs of the furtive, big cats are seldom seen. Coyotes and small forest animals live here as well. You are most likely to see small rodents, as they attempt to secure food from you in the established campgrounds. Don't feed them. Over 1,500 plant species have been identified in the park. And of course there are hundreds of different birds, reptiles, and amphibians. You will likely hear tree frogs at night while you are trying to sleep. You may be awakened at dawn by the eerie, haunting cry of a loon, if you're lucky. In many areas, this sound is considered the seal of wilderness.

Because Ross Lake, and the Skagit River flowing into it, are in steep snow country, many avalanches occur during winter and early spring. Avalanches rip out trees and undergrowth, which are then carried down into or near the water. At least for Ross Lake, the result is a fair amount of flotsam (or floating wood) in the water. This is of little concern to the kayaker who, traveling slowly, has plenty of time to spot driftwood, and can easily maneuver around

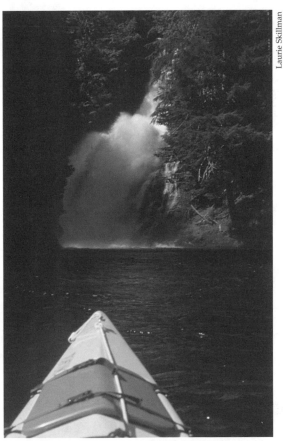

Laurie Skillman

After snowmelt, Arctic Creek plunges into Ross Lake with a thunderous roar

obstacles. This is not the case for powerboaters, who must exercise great care on Ross. It is not uncommon to see whole trees floating in the lake near the upper end.

Camping at the Hozomeen Campground is free, with sites available on a first-come, first-served basis. Campground facilities—including the boat camps along the lake—are unusually well maintained here. Because ranger boat patrols are frequently on the water, make sure you follow the rules and obtain a boat-camping permit. The plus side to this extensive patrol effort is that help is available if needed, and adhering to the rules preserves the wilderness nature of the area. Remember that random camping along shore is not allowed. It is easy to promote good sanitary practices here: just use the toilets at the various camps, whether you are visiting for a few minutes, or are staying there.

Trip Description

Launch at Hozomeen, and paddle south along the east shore of Ross Lake. As soon as you are out on the water, a glance over your left shoulder reveals Hozomeen Mountain, rearing glaciated, granite spires skyward to 8,068 feet. You will see these rounded spires again when you are farther south on the lake. For the first 2 miles, you are heading slightly southwest, and then southeast as you round the broad point at the base of Little Jackass Mountain. If you launched from the campground area, you will pass the main launching ramp, dock, and small boathouse within 0.5 mile, and then the Park Service maintenance dock within another 0.5 mile. Construction and maintenance on the boat camps is handled from this dock.

After 2 miles from launch Silver Creek Campground will be on your right, along the west shore of the lake. Notice that Silver Creek has deposited a considerable amount of alluvial material, forming a narrow band of gently sloping shore here. For the most part, this alluvial bench is densely covered with alder, cottonwood, and mixed conifers. Almost due west 6 miles up Silver Creek is Silver Lake (not to be confused with the Silver Lake in BC), fed by glaciers on the north slopes of 8,980-foot Mount Spickard. There is no trail.

Rounding Little Jackass Mountain, you'll see Jack Point to the south on the east shore (4 miles from launch). Ross Lake in this section is less then a mile wide. Dense timber on both shores extends to the water, and there are few—if any—good places to land. In the easternmost curve of the bay south of Jack Point is Boundary Bay Campground, one of six boat camps that are designated group camps. Here, you are 5.5 miles from launch.

One mile south of Jack Point, on the opposite (west) shore, is a broad, unnamed point toward which you can paddle if the weather is good. One mile south of the unnamed point on the west shore is Little Beaver

Campground (6 miles from launch). There is a small cabin at this camp. Sites are scattered about on rounded wooded knobs, and there is an excellent new dock. Steel, bear-proof food boxes have been installed here.

Little Beaver Trail, which joins other major trails to the west in the interior of North Cascades National Park, terminates in this camp at Ross Lake. The trail closely follows Little Beaver Creek for 13 miles to Whatcom Pass. Here, Ross Lake juts west into the cramped canyon of Little Beaver Creek, creating a narrow estuary for several hundred feet. Maidenhair ferns adorn granite boulders, and conifers bonsai'd by harsh conditions grow horizontally from cliffs before curving skyward. It is a great place to sit in your boat and observe.

Paddle south 0.9 mile from Little Beaver Creek along the west shore to Arctic Creek. During spring and early summer Arctic Creek delivers its considerable flow to Ross Lake in a thunderous waterfall, which begins as a series of cascades hidden in timber several hundred feet above. The last 75 feet is a free fall to the lake's edge, a sight to see. Another 0.9 mile south of Arctic Creek, No Name Creek reaches Ross Lake, also via cataracts, but with a lesser flow mostly hidden by foliage.

One mile directly opposite Arctic Creek on the east shore is a prominent point, around which Ross Lake bends slightly east of south. Desolation Peak (6,102') lies 2 miles east from the point. Cat Island, the destination on this trip, has been in sight since you were north of Arctic Creek. It is the rounded, wooded island near the east shore. From Arctic Creek, you can paddle directly east across Ross Lake and then go south to Cat Island, not a bad idea if the wind looks like it might kick up. If conditions are favorable, head directly to Cat Island from Arctic Creek, a distance of 2 miles.

Nearly circular and some two hundred yards across, Cat Island rises 40 feet above lake level. A light stand of conifers covers the island and offers shade. The dock is on the north end of the island. There are four campsites; the two on the west side of the island are close to the water and would be best for kayak camping, since you can pull your boat up on shore near your camp. The other two sites, accessible from the dock, are located on knolls in the center of the island and are elevated nearly 40 feet above the dock. There are tables and fire rings at each site. Pit toilets are located at the northwest end of the island, near the sign identifying the camp.

The Desolation Trail to Desolation Peak follows along the east shore of Ross Lake, branching from the East Bank Trail at Lightning Creek, 1 mile south of Cat Island. A suspension bridge, which carries the trail across the interesting, narrow estuary of Lightning Creek, is clearly seen from Cat Island. It is worth the paddle down there just to experience the estuary. This trip ends at Cat Island. To return to Hozomeen, retrace the route that brought you here. If conditions are calm, you might consider paddling back along the shore you didn't see on the way to Cat Island.

Additional or Alternate Trips

With 19 campsites on Ross Lake, obviously there are many possible trip combinations. Remember that you must have a boat-camp permit for each night you camp on the shore, and this limits you to a specific camp for each night. By planning your trip during the week rather than over a weekend, you will have a good chance to secure the camps and days you prefer. It may be necessary to stay two nights in one camp, or paddle farther than you would like in order to reach a camp where sites are available, but—with planning and by remaining flexible—you can devise a leisurely paddle of several days on Ross Lake. Rangers know the lake and the camps well, and will often have suggestions. Also, consider mixing a day of hiking with your paddle trip if you must stay in one camp two nights. Hike right from camp if it has access to one of the trails. Or you could paddle to a trail access and hike for that day, paddling back to your designated camp at day's end.

Another option is to begin your trip from the south at Ross Lake Resort, using the resort's portage service. Doing so eliminates the long drive through British Columbia to Hozomeen. Once on Ross Lake, plan your trip beginning at the resort, as available permits allow, just as if you began at Hozomeen on the north end.

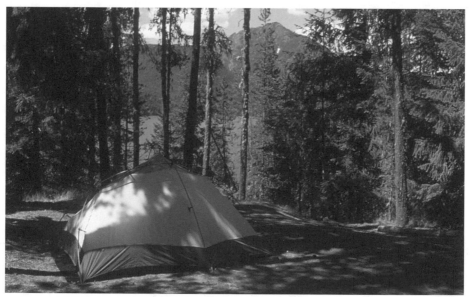

A view of Ross Lake from the hilltop campsite on Cat Island

Campsite Descriptions (south to north)

Green Point—On a sparsely wooded knoll on the west shore, and just 0.5 mile from Ross Lake Resort (1 mile from Ross Lake Dam; 22 miles from Hozomeen). Seven sites, hiking trail, dock.

Cougar Island—On a 200-yard-wide island, 2 miles from Ross Lake Dam and 21 miles from Hozomeen. There are two sites and a dock.

Roland Point—On a small peninsula on the east shore, with entrance behind point to the east. Sheltered bay, but only one wooded site, no dock. Ross Lake Dam is 4 miles distant and Hozomeen is 19 miles.

Big Beaver—On the west shore at the estuary of Big Beaver Creek, which occupies a sizable gorge terminating in clifflike slopes and timbered flats. Big Beaver, 4 miles from the dam and 19 miles from Hozomeen, has seven sites, a hiking trail, and a dock.

McMillan—Located on the north side of the east-shore peninsula from Roland Point. There are three sites here, with a group camp, and a dock. It is 5.5 miles to the dam and 17.5 miles to Hozomeen. Good protection from the south here, but open to the north.

Spencer's Camp—On a broad point which juts into the lake, forming small bays on either side. Good protection from north and south here, but only two sites and a dock. The dam is 6 miles distant, and it is 17 miles to Hozomeen. Views are fantastic from this camp.

May Creek—The single site here is on a rounded point, in heavy timber, and well protected from the north but not so well from the south. Located at the small waterfall where May Creek enters, the site's backdrop are cliffs and a slope which rises to above timberline a mile inland. There is a hiking trail and a dock. The dam is 6.5 miles; Hozomeen 16.5.

Rainbow Point—In a small bight, with dock and trail. The three sites are 7.5 miles from the dam and 15.5 miles from Hozomeen. Sites are in a stand of old-growth timber.

Devils Junction—A single site here, with dock. Near the junction with East Bank Trail and the trail east to Devils Dome. Good protection from the south at this timbered spot 10.5 miles from the dam; 12.5 miles from Hozomeen.

Ten Mile Island—There are three sites here, with no dock. The island is a few hundred yards across, with the sites at water's edge. The dam is 11 miles distant, and it is 12 miles to Hozomeen.

Dry Creek & Ponderosa—These camps are on opposite sides of the same rocky peninsula, with four sites on the former and two on the latter. There is no dock at either. It is 12 miles to the dam, and 11 to Hozomeen. While shading timber is sparse, there is sufficient for shade, and the view is good.

Lodgepole—Located 12.5 miles from the dam and 10.5 from Hozomeen, this camp is situated in a patch of lodgepole pines, just a couple of feet above the water level. There are three sites and access to a hiking trail, but no dock.

Lightning Creek Boat Camp—Lightning Creek Horse Camp, located a short distance away on the south side of the bridge over Lightning Creek, is not intended for boat campers. The boat camp is 13.5 miles north of the dam, and 9.5 miles from Hozomeen. There are six sites here, with bear boxes, trail access, and a dock. There are lots of deciduous trees around the campground which turn color in the fall. Don't miss paddling up the narrow cove where Lightning Creek enters.

Cat Island—Four sites, with dock. The dam is 14.5 miles, while Hozomeen is 8.5 miles distant.

Little Beaver—On a series of rounded knolls on the west shore, at the entrance of Little Beaver Creek. Five sites here have access to a hiking trail, and there is a dock. 17 miles to the dam, while Hozomeen is 6 miles distant.

Boundary Bay—There are three sites at this group camp, located on one of the steepest shorelines of all the camps. The dam is 17.5 miles distant, and it is 5.5 miles to Hozomeen. There is no dock.

Silver Creek—One of the four camps on the west shore of Ross Lake. Four sites here, and a dock. It is 21 miles to the dam, and 2 miles to Hozomeen.

All of the campgrounds mentioned above have pit toilets, tables, fire rings, and superb scenery.

Contacts
Ross Lake Resort

The only facility on Ross Lake, situated near the dam for the past 49 years, the resort is unique in offering floating cabins for guests in addition to outboard-boat and kayak rentals. The resort provides a portage service to place boaters on Ross Lake. Not accessible by road, the resort is reached by taking the Seattle City Light tugboat, either at 8:30 a.m. or 3:30 p.m. daily, across Diablo Lake to Ross Dam. To take your paddle boat, launch on Diablo Lake and paddle east to Ross Dam. By prior arrangement the resort vehicle will meet you. Alternatively, you can also walk the 2 miles to Ross Lake Resort, from milepost 134 on Hwy. 20. Call (206) 386-4437 for more information, and portaging or rental arrangements.

North Cascades National Park (May through September)
Wilderness Information Center
728 Ranger Station Rd.
Marblemount, WA 98267
(360) 873-4500 ext. 39

North Cascades National Park (October through April)
2105 Highway 20
Sedro-Woolley, WA 98284
(360) 856-5700

We launched at Hozomeen early, while the loons were still calling. Quietly, so as not to disturb the other camps, we slipped our double kayak into the calm water and paddled away. Ross Lake was awakening, the glassy surface just beginning to show a few riffles. Within a few hundred yards we were far enough out that the surrounding peaks no longer hid our view of the backcountry, and the rounded, glaciated spires of Hozomeen Mountain became visible to the east.

A layering of low clouds, foglike, hung over the lake, partly obscuring the peaks around us. We looked at the timbered shorelines, and the layered clouds, and it was easy to imagine we were again paddling in Misty Fjords off Alaska's Inland Passage. Then the clouds broke and we could see Neve Glacier, cupped inside the jagged ridges of Snowfield Peak far to the south. As the clouds dissipated, a breeze arrived, propelling us southward.

About the time we could make out Cat Island, a deep roar, rumbling from the west shore, caught our attention. We swung the bow toward the sound, and soon we saw mist and spray shooting out over the lake from behind a rocky point. As our angle of approach changed, the mist became prismatic, with rainbow tints implying a peace that the roar belies. There is nothing peaceful about the winds accompanying the waterfall. A wet spray, created as the falls emphatically meets the lake surface, blasts out across the water. Dripping with spray after playing in the current, we left the spectacle to resume our paddle.

Gracing a rocky point, a tall shoreline snag terminated in a large osprey nest. The quick, swooping of a kingfisher marked its flight past us to an overhanging limb. Flying higher, its neck curved back in a question mark, a blue heron crossed the lake. A loon, fishing near shore, eyed us nervously and then dove. Minutes later we arrived at Cat Island.

We took the campsite at the top of the hill. With no sign of clouds now, the sun blazed down, making us grateful for the shade proffered around camp. As we were alternately immersed in our surroundings and books, the day wore on; we decided to take a quick dip. The effects of frigid Ross Lake water were immediate, and so was the end of our swimming.

A deer walked through camp. Strange that a deer would live on such a small island used by campers all summer. Then we observed that the deer's coat was as wet as our swimsuits. She had just come to visit from the mainland.

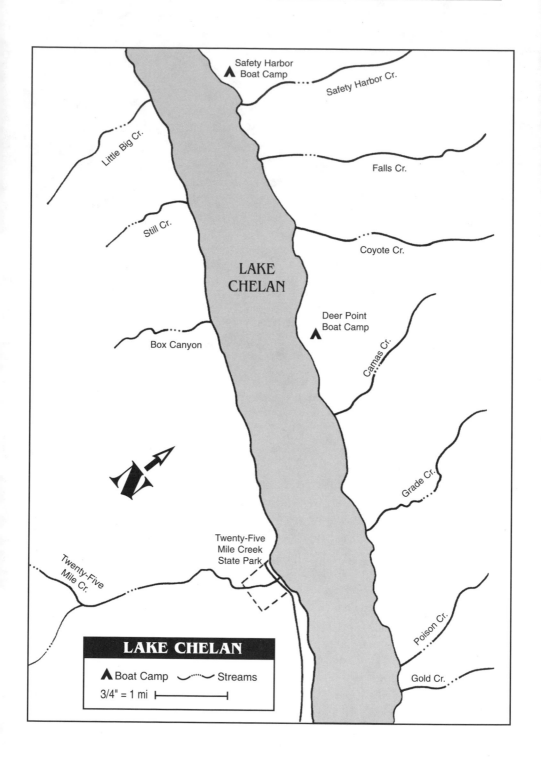

Washington

Chapter 4

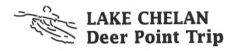 **LAKE CHELAN**
Deer Point Trip

Trip Details

Distance:	7 miles
Time:	3 hours paddling
Rating:	Easy to Moderate
Maps:	USGS 7.5-min: *Stormy Mountain* and *South Navarre Peak*

Summary and Highlights

This trip is short, given the possibilities on Lake Chelan. The launch is from Twenty-Five Mile Creek State Park, and the paddle is a leisurely trip across the lake, then north to Deer Point. This also makes a good day trip, if you don't want to camp overnight. Crossing Chelan provides a good taste of both the size and vagaries of this large inland, glacier-gouged lake. At times the lake is mild, exhibiting a glassy-calm surface. At other times, breezes that blow down-lake spring up suddenly, keeping kayakers on their toes.

Deer Point is a pleasant spot, with sites sprinkled over a low, rocky point. There are gravel beaches on each side of the point when the water level is at full pool. The floating dock is on the south side of the point, in a small cove that provides excellent protection from down-lake winds. Much of the point is timbered with conifers, in contrast to other abruptly rising, west-facing slopes along this stretch of lake, which are clad customarily in dry grass, with occasional trees and patches of brush. The five sites at Deer Point have tables and fire rings. Pit toilets are provided.

When to go: Lake Chelan does not freeze over during normal winters. So, you can paddle there any time of the year. Spring, summer, and fall are most pleasant, with May through September being the best in terms of temperature. However, spring is noted for windy conditions and, on this lake, that is a major consideration. Residents at Chelan note that the lake is often calm during the hot days of summer. Lake Chelan hosts a large development of vacation homes, which bring significant boating activity to the south end of the lake. Twenty-Five Mile Creek State Park is about 20 miles by water north of the populated end of Lake Chelan. Because nearly all summer homes are south of the park, when you paddle north from there, you rapidly leave behind casual recreational users. To achieve the greatest seclusion during your paddle, try to schedule your trip midweek, particularly right after the weekend. By Thursday or Friday, weekend usage increases again.

Hazards: Lake Chelan waters are so cold that prolonged immersion is sure to bring on hypothermia. Since being unprotected in the water for even a short period can cause you to loose the use of muscles in your extremities, be cautious and paddle only when conditions are well within your comfort and experience range.

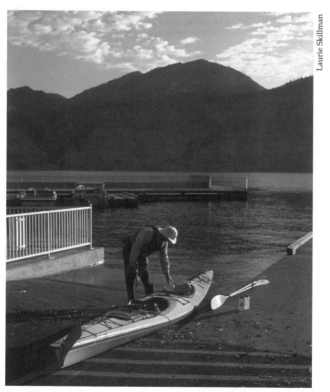

Launching at Twenty-Five Mile Creek SP positions the paddler for up-lake exploration

Wind, of course, causes waves, which can build up to a point where paddle boats capsize. This is the case on all large bodies of water, but is especially a factor on Lake Chelan. The 55-mile-long lake provides a perfect channel for relatively unobstructed winds. In addition, the canyons of several major drainage systems intersect the lake, providing conduits for cold, gravity winds. An area roughly in the middle of Lake Chelan known as "The Straits" can be especially windy. Watch for wind signs on the water horizon, and, if dangerous conditions occur, go ashore and wait for improvement.

How to Get There

Lake Chelan lies off Highway 97 immediately northwest of the town of Chelan, very near the geographical center of Washington. Hwy. 97 Alternate runs right through the town. From Chelan drive west along Hwy. 97 Alt., and in 4 miles turn right (north) and proceed along the lakeshore road to Twenty-Five Mile Creek State Park.

Area Features, Background, and Tips

The North Cascades rose to their present heights over millions of years. Today the uplifting has stopped, and the mountains are being gradually eroded away; you needn't hurry, because this is a slow process. Much of the rock in this section of the Cascades is gneiss, a metamorphosed volcanic sediment. Other rocks are granite, formed when molten magma deep beneath the earth's crust flowed upward along fault lines without reaching the surface, solidifying and cooling slowly. Where molten rock did reach the surface, a volcano was formed.

While erosion from water helped shape the major landforms, glaciers were the main sculptors. As uplift began, water in the form of streams began contouring the surface, flowing seaward. As the mountains became higher, what had been rain turned into snow, forming snowpacks and, eventually, glaciers. While following streambeds for the most part, these glaciers often cut their own canyons as well. Over millenniums glaciers advanced and receded many times over the valley that is today Lake Chelan. The last retreat some 17,000 years ago left a valley scoured and quarried to a depth of 600 feet below sea level. Water-borne sediments from the Stehekin River and major tributaries have since filled this canyon to 440 feet below sea level. With a depth of 1,541 feet, Chelan is the third-deepest lake in the U.S.

Glacial signs are clearly visible as you paddle. Note the remains of lateral moraines on the north shore, far above the present lake level. Since glacial ice was more than a mile thick here, the tops of many lakeside peaks present smooth, rounded, glaciated profiles. When the glaciers were melting away from Lake Chelan, the lake outlet at what is now the town of Chelan was still deeply covered. The inflow of water raised the lake hundreds of feet above the present level, seeking an outlet to the sea. Full to overflowing, the lake cut Knapp's Coulee, a new outlet to the Columbia River. A similar incident incised Navarre Coulee. Both outlets became high and dry after the ice dam at Chelan broke, allowing lake runoff to again flow to the Columbia via the Chelan River.

When the first Euro-white explorers were sizing up the country for the fur trade, natives had been living in the Lake Chelan area for centuries. An Indian village with perhaps 100 inhabitants was located near the present town of Chelan. Hunting and gathering was good, with game in the valleys along the river, fish in the lake and streams, and edible plants and berries everywhere during their seasons. As pressure from settlers increased, a reservation was first created and later nullified by Congress in 1886. Yet, Native Americans were allowed to gain title to land in the area, which some did. Others moved to the Colville Reservation near Okanagan, Washington.

Miners prospected the area beginning in the 1880s, particularly in the Stehekin and Railroad Creek areas. Mines were established, and operated for varying periods of time. Perhaps most significant was the Holden Mine, about 12 miles up Railroad Creek from the lake. The ore body was discovered in 1896, and figured prominently in copper production in Washington. The mine was finally closed in 1957, after having played an important economic role in the region. The railroad planned for the creek of the same name never materialized. Lucerne, at the confluence of Railroad Creek and Lake Chelan, functioned as a sort of lakeside mining camp. Today, the landing is a staging stop for visitors going to Holden and those headed for wilderness areas in the North Cascades.

There being no roads the length of Lake Chelan, freight and commerce to the mines was by boat from the growing town of Chelan. To supply the mines, homesteaders moved in and began farming various crops. Irrigation was needed for this, since Chelan is located in the arid "rain shadow" of the Cascades. Flumes and ditches were constructed, bringing water from tributary creeks along the north shore of Lake Chelan. Because the last of these old works was abandoned in the early 1970s, since that time irrigation water has been pumped from the lake for the considerable agriculture in the area.

While the mines were active, the town of Stehekin became popular as a resort. Vacationers were numerous enough to support a splendid, 100-visitor Victorian hotel at Stehekin, even though it could be reached only by boat. Several other hotels were built nearby, as the miners and tourists required more accommodations.

By 1926, plans had progressed to raise the level of Lake Chelan 20 feet with a dam for hydroelectric generation. The Victorian hotel at Stehekin, as well as many other structures along the lakeshore, came down just before inundation. Unfortunately, Native American sites along the natural shoreline were also flooded. Today, the lake is at the full-pool elevation of 1,100 feet during most of the summer season. Normal variation is 10-18', with the lowest levels just before spring runoff begins.

Today, access to the upper lake is by boat or floatplane. A road has been constructed from Chelan to Twenty-Five Mile Creek along the south shore of the lake. In Depression days, CCC crews constructed a trail from Twenty-Five Mile Creek nearly 4 miles up-lake to Box Canyon. But, other than very occasional pieces of private property acquired from mining claims, that is the extent of development until one moves up-lake to Lucerne, and on to Stehekin. This lack of access points is one factor that makes Lake Chelan appealing for a kayak trip.

If ever the adjective "fjordlike" applies, it does to Lake Chelan. Much of the shoreline is precipitous cliffs that plunge far below the water's surface. Only occasional flatter, alluvial plains are present, notably where major creeks run into the lake. Both shores, from Chelan up-lake to Twenty-Five Mile Creek are characterized by seasonal grasses and undergrowth, the signature of semiarid climatic conditions. A few miles northwest of Twenty-Five Mile Creek, the south shore with its north-facing slope is moist enough to support conifer

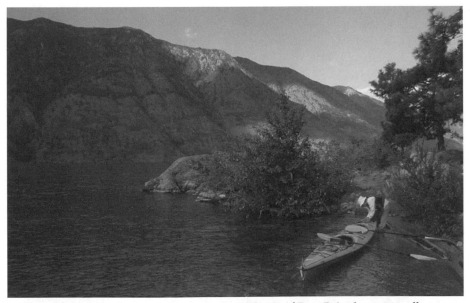

Though cramped, this Chelan camp 0.25 mile northwest of Deer Point boat camp offers a tent site, shade, wind protection, and spectacular views

growth. The opposite shore, which faces south and dries out more quickly, only supports scattered conifers.

Generous flows from tributaries early in the season make stream water easily obtainable at that time. Lake water can be used for drinking, provided it is treated, filtered, or boiled. While camping is permitted along shore on public land, most of the good camping areas have been developed by the Park Service and Forest Service into boat-in campgrounds. A dock-use permit is required to use the boat-in campgrounds on Lake Chelan. These are obtainable at the state parks, and also at the ranger station in Chelan. Roadside camping is available at the two state parks on Lake Chelan (see Contacts, later in this chapter).

Trip Description

Launch at the Twenty-Five Mile Creek State Park ramp and paddle due north 1.2 miles to the north shore of Lake Chelan. Do not set out on this crossing unless the conditions (and the conditions you think will occur a half-hour later) are within your experience level. The cabins you see along the north shore are on those one-time mining claims. Notice that all are accessed by boat. Then paddle northwest 2 miles along the north shore to Deer Point. The point is easily spotted, not only because the rocky point projects into the lake a couple of hundred feet, but because there is a dense patch of conifers upon it, contrasting with adjoining slopes in this area.

There is a nice floating dock at Deer Point, serving five tent sites with fire rings and tables. Two toilets here assure proper sanitation. The cove south of the point provides excellent shelter from down-lake wind waves, and there is a small gravel beach. A longer gravel beach graces the opposite side of the point. Lower water levels may expose more beaches, or strand them well above the water.

Of interest is a second point just up-lake (north) from Deer Point. However undeveloped, there is room for at least one camp here, and—while there is no dock or toilet—a gravel beach makes access easy when the lake is full. Campers using undeveloped sites should pack out all waste.

From Deer Point, return to Twenty-Five Mile Creek. If the wind is calm, you can cross over (head south) to the south shore of Lake Chelan, then paddle east to Twenty-Five Mile Creek. If you choose this route, you will see remains of the old Box Canyon CCC Trail along the shore.

Additional Trips

With more than 30 miles of lake stretching northwest into wilderness, there are many trip combinations that you can make, depending upon your available time, your experience, and other factors. Here are some suggestions:

Since prevailing winds are down-lake, some paddlers may want to take their boats to Stehekin on the north end of the lake, and paddle back. The northern two thirds of the lake can be paddled leisurely in three days. To accomplish this, ship your boat for a small charge on one of the two companies running freight barges weekly on Lake Chelan. You will need to take the daily passenger ferry to Stehekin, since the freight barges do not carry passengers. If you embark on the ferry at Fields Point, north of Chelan and just south of Twenty-Five Mile Creek, you will not only pay a lesser fare, but be able to put your car in their huge parking lot for a small fee. Better ship your duffel on the barge, or keep it less than the 75 lbs. per person allowed on the ferry (see Contacts later in this chapter).

Campsite Descriptions (south to north)

It is easy to plan a longer trip to one or more of the other boat-in campgrounds. Here is a list noting the facilities provided and the distance from launch at Twenty-Five Mile Creek State Park followed by the distance to Stehekin. If there are feasible landing sites and possible campsites between the boat-in campgrounds, they are noted also. Descriptions of undeveloped sites are flagged (below) by indented text.

Deer Point—(3.5 miles from launch at Twenty-Five Mile Creek; 28.5 miles to Stehekin) A good floating dock in a small cove with protection from the north makes this a welcome campground. There are five sites with fire rings and tables. Two toilets are located at this north-shore location.

Safety Harbor— (7 miles; 25 miles) Great shelter from both up-lake and down-lake winds makes this a popular site, with a floating dock for access to four sites, two tables, two fire rings, and a toilet. Its location is on the north shore in a small cove at the inflow of Harbor Creek. Abrupt cliffs just up-lake plunge beneath the surface making the water near shore quite deep.

A small cove at the entrance to nearby Coyote Creek, on the north shore, provides some wind protection. It is possible to go ashore here, but landing would be on boulders and camping would be problematic. *This is a site for emergencies only.*

Big Creek—(9; 23) On the south shore, this campground boasts a shelter, four tent sites with tables and fire rings, and two toilets have been installed. The dock is stationary, and there is a gravel beach. The shoreline here is more heavily timbered.

Corral Creek—(10; 22) Expect good shelter from wind from either direction at the floating dock. There are four tent sites, three tables, two fire rings, and a toilet here, on the south shore.

At Big Goat Creek, on the north shore directly north of Corral Creek, there is a gravel beach in a small indented cove. It would be possible to land at this location if needed, and also at Little Goat Creek just up-lake.

Graham Harbor—(13; 19) Located on a knobby glaciated point, this spot has a floating dock with protection from down-lake wind. It should also be possible to land on the gravel beach here. There are five tent sites, seven tables, six fire rings, and two toilets at this west-shore camp.

Graham Harbor Creek—(13; 19) This nearby timbered site on the west shore has a shelter, five tent sites—each with a table and fire ring—and there are two toilets. The dock here is stationary.

A small alluvial fan on the east shore just south of Canoe Creek will permit landing. The buildings at Canoe Creek itself are on private land.

Prince Creek—(18; 14) This creek is quite large, and has built a sizable alluvial fan that results in a gravel landing beach. There are four tent sites, each with a table and fire ring. There are two toilets at this camp, which the dock makes accessible year-round. Protection from down-lake wind is good at this east-shore location.

Domke Falls—(21; 11) This camp is 200 yards up-lake from the falls on the west shore. Located on a rounded knoll, it has five tent sites, seven tables, six fire rings, two toilets, and a floating dock. Domke Creek drains Domke Lake, a mile-long glacial lake 1.5 miles northwest. The lake and camps around it are reached by trail from Lucerne.

Refrigerator Harbor—(24; 8) There are several docks at this site, and some facilities here have been leased to a yacht club. This was the original mining company landing. Lucerne is located on the opposite side of Railroad Creek. Refrigerator Harbor is accessible year-round, with four tent sites—each with a table and fire ring—and two toilets. Down-lake wind protection is good at this west-shore camp.

Lucerne—(24.5; 7.5) This is the facility that once served the mines at Holden. A major dock allows for freight transfer and the daily ferry stops here. There are buildings and other facilities. Lucerne offers gravel beaches when the lake is full. The Forest Service camp is located adjacent to the guard station and has two tables with fire rings, and two toilets.

Moore Point—(27; 5) This camp on the east shore is just south of Fish Creek and adjacent to private land on this prominent point. The facilities consist of a shelter, four tables and fire rings, and two toilets. The dock is stationary.

From Wolverine Creek, just opposite Moore Point, the west shore is heavily timbered to the upper end of the lake. South of here, the coniferous forest has been spotty—with evidence of old forest fires. The east shore, with south- and west-facing exposures, is much less hospitable to coniferous forest.

Flick Creek—(29.5; 2.5) on the east shore and **Manley Wham** just opposite on the west shore are camps located within the Lake Chelan National Recreation Area. There are four sites at Manley Wham, and a single site at Flick Creek. Both camps are approximately 2.5 miles south of Stehekin. Other camps at the head of the lake are at Stehekin, Purple Point, and Weaver Point.

Other Area Activities

In Chelan: Besides the obvious watersports, there are over 200 miles of trails available in the Chelan Ranger District (see Contacts). Mountain bikers will discover many back roads, and will be especially challenged by the dirt road to the top of Chelan Butte. This steep road is passable by car, and the view of Lake Chelan and the Columbia River from the 3,835-foot summit is worth the trip. Keep your vehicle in low gear both ways. Hang gliding is popular from this summit.

Almost a must is a trip on the Lady of the Lake ferry, which daily makes a round trip to Stehekin. Even if you have kayaked on much of Lake Chelan, the ferry trip will give you a different, effortless perspective of not only the lake but its surroundings.

In Stehekin: Many hiking trails are available from the Stehekin area, which lies inside North Cascades National Park. A small bus plies the 12 or so miles of road leading up the Stehekin River from the settlement, giving access to notable, 312'-high Rainbow Falls, as well as campgrounds and trailheads within the park. This closed-road system is completely isolated from the outside by many miles of rough terrain. Visit the Golden West Visitor Center in Stehekin, a National Park facility offering exhibits, information, maps, and books. Self-guided walking tours will further acquaint you with the history of Stehekin.

Contacts

For back-country permits, dock permits, and boating and hiking information contact:

U.S. Forest Service/National Park Service
Chelan Ranger District
PO Box 189
Chelan, WA 98816
(509) 682-2576

Permits for using Forest Service and Park Service docks are also available from various retailers in Chelan. For Stehekin information contact:

National Park Service
PO Box 7

Stehekin, WA 98852
(509) 682-2549

The Lady of the Lake passenger ferries are operated by:
Lake Chelan Boat Co.
PO Box 186
Chelan, WA 98816
(509) 682-2224

Barging of paddle boats to Stehekin is provided by Lake Chelan Boat Co. Other barges also ply the lake on varying schedules; inquire at the boat company.

Washington State Park reservations, including those at **Twenty-Five Mile Creek State Park** and **Lake Chelan State Park** (both on Lake Chelan) can be made by calling: (800) 452-5687.

The Lake Chelan Chamber of Commerce is another good source of information. Contact them at:
PO Box 216
Chelan, WA 98816
(800) 424-3526

Today was calm as we paddled out from the launch area at Twenty-Five Mile Creek State Park. What a contrast from a few weeks earlier, when a springtime low-pressure system kicked up 3'-high wind waves on Lake Chelan in this very spot, keeping us off the water for several days. We weren't even able to launch on that trip, but today we couldn't ask for a better morning.

Even so, we kept a weather eye to the northwest as we began crossing Chelan. Sure enough, a dark line soon appeared on the water horizon, and gradually extended toward us. But the dark line did not progress into whiteness signifing whitecaps, and all that affected us were a few diminishing waves. By the time we made the north shore, the wind had become spotty, allowing patches of glassy-calm. We swung west, gliding easily along the shore.

A scattering of cabins along this shore surprised us. But reached only by boat, their appearance conveyed that the owners must value privacy and have a high level of caring for the lake. Soon we were past the farthest structure and moving easily up-lake. Close to shore the water took on the emerald cast that comes just before you can make out details on the bottom. Beyond these shallower spots the water reverted to the authoritarian indigo of great depth.

A string of small clouds out of the west now announced their presence with a scattering of large raindrops. First a hiss, they increased in frequency until the water surface jumped to a staccato roar. Instantly drenched, we stopped paddling and watched the water running off our spray skirts in rivulets. The shower persisted for a while, slowed—sounding like a Peruvian rainstick, and then stopped as suddenly as it began.

An occasional gull flew past. We spotted deer ashore, browsing on buckbrush and some volunteer apple seedlings left over from earlier days. We paddled on leisurely toward the timber-studded projection of shore that we knew was Deer Point. A single powerboat was moored at the dock, its occupants sitting around a tent pitched just above it with a beautiful view of the lake. We opted to be alone, and so paddled a few hundred yards past Deer Point to a smaller point we'd seen.

In spite of the midsummer season, no one was at this secondary point. A large granite boulder with an accompanying pine tree graced the spot, offering a flat area more than sufficient to pitch our tent. Prior users had erected a windbreak from driftwood, which would be helpful if the wind increased in the afternoon. We would, of course, be without facilities if we camped here, but that was a small sacrifice for this storybook site. We popped loose spray skirts and headed in to the sheltered, fine-gravel beach.

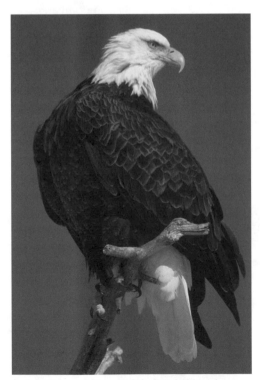

Subsisting mainly on a fish diet, bald eagles can be found around bodies of water—especially in the northern states

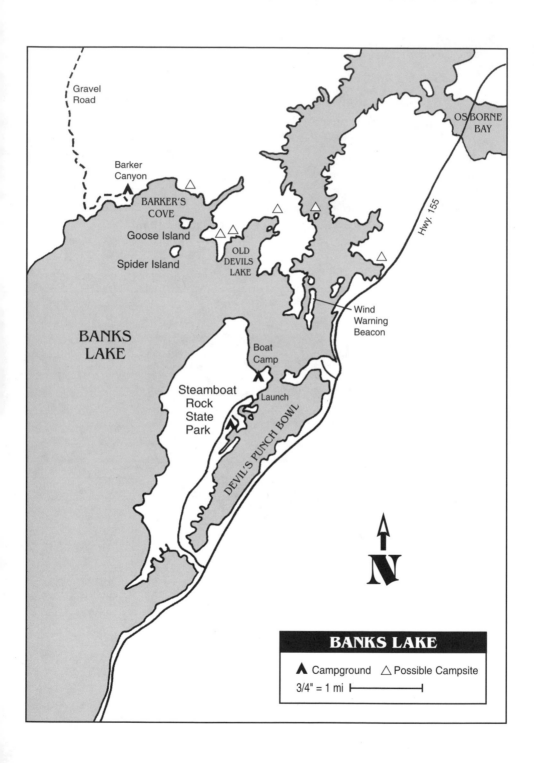

Gravel
Road

Barker
Canyon

BARKER'S
COVE

Goose Island

Spider Island

OSBORNE
BAY

Hwy. 155

OLD
DEVILS
LAKE

Wind
Warning
Beacon

BANKS
LAKE

Boat
Camp

Steamboat
Rock
State
Park

Launch

DEVIL'S PUNCH BOWL

N

BANKS LAKE

▲ Campground   △ Possible Campsite
3/4" = 1 mi

Washington

Chapter 5

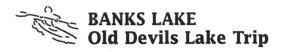

BANKS LAKE
Old Devils Lake Trip

Trip Details

Distance:	6 miles
Time:	3 hours paddling
Rating:	Easy to Moderate
Maps:	USGS 7.5-min: *Steamboat Rock SE*, *Steamboat Rock SW*, *Barker Canyon*, and *Electric City*;or the excellent chart *Banks Lake*, Washington, available from Northwest Map Service, W 525 Sprague Ave., Spokane, WA 99204 (509) 455-6981

Summary and Highlights

Picture a high-desert lake where you can paddle beneath majestic, lichen-covered cliffs towering hundreds of feet above your kayak. A few willows occupy pockets along the shore and occasional, stunted cottonwoods provide a little shade. But the overview is of water expanses, sagebrush, and the ever-present basaltic cliffs. This is wild but accessible Banks Lake, just waiting to be paddled.

Mention Grand Coulee and you conjure up images of the dam. The famous dam is not in the Grand Coulee at all, but on the Columbia River in east-central Washington. The Grand Coulee is actually a flood channel, cut when glacial ice dams blocked the Columbia River waterway and diverted the flow into a new channel. Sudden release of Lake Missoula in Montana, when another ice dam gave way, further gouged the coulee. This huge flood channel is today the site of Banks Lake, created by the Bureau of Reclamation as part of an irrigation project in conjunction with Grand Coulee Dam on the Columbia River.

Pumped by a portion of the electricity generated by the powerhouse at Grand Coulee Dam, Columbia River water fills Banks Lake. At 1,570' elevation, the Banks Lake Reservoir is high enough for gravity to carry irrigation water through canals and natural channels to vast agricultural acreages in central Washington. That the water level avoids the wild fluctuations of most reservoirs and varies only 5 feet is a big plus to kayakers. Paddling on Banks Lake is like boating on a natural lake with a nearly unchanging shoreline.

Banks Lake's 28-mile length fills the coulee bottom, which runs north-northeast and south-southwest. The northern portion of the lake exhibits the most striking features and is 5 miles wide at its broadest. Ever-present here are the near-vertical walls of Grand Coulee itself, rising up 700 feet from the lake to the level of the broad plateau from which the coulee was torn. A number of small, fun-to-explore islets dot the northern portion, and there are numerous narrow channels and inlets adding interest to this kayak trip. Oddly enough, much of the shoreline and many islets are granite, not basalt like the cliffs of the coulee walls.

Steamboat Rock is actually a 3-mile-long by 1-mile-wide peninsula, at the widest part of the lake. The rock escaped being torn away by the torrent that carved Grand Coulee because the basalt forming the peninsula was harder and more resistant than surrounding formations, which are no longer there. Protected by jagged cliffs, the northern third of the peninsula juts—mesa-like—700 feet above the water. The southern two thirds of the peninsula is a wildlife refuge, and also the site of Steamboat Rock State Park. The park camping areas are verdant oases at the water's edge, in contrast to the stark, dry surroundings. The state park is a convenient starting point for a paddle trip on the lake.

Averaging 1.5 miles in width, the lake's southern portion seems crowded between the cliffs on either shore. Ambitious paddlers may want to explore the 15-mile length of this narrowest half of Banks Lake. But kayaking anywhere on Banks gives the paddler a feeling of moving back in time. When you realize what caused the landscape all around you—when you visualize the huge flood torrents carving away cubic miles of rock—you feel insignificant and awed. Knowing this was both a home and a natural larder for Native Americans over the millenniums imparts another aura, as you glide by the same lichen-studded cliffs those earlier people saw.

When to go: Spring, when temperatures have warmed somewhat, is a good time to visit Banks Lake to see late-migrant waterfowl. When present in the spring, they add their numbers to the local resident ducks, Canada geese, herons, eagles, and occasional prairie falcons. Keep in mind that conditions in early spring include sudden temperature swings and the possibility of more wind than you would prefer. Summer is warm in the Grand Coulee. During periods of high atmospheric pressure, its comparatively low elevation increases heating. During these hot spells, the air can be still and the lake glassy. Because the desert environment is lacking in shade, while you might have calm water, you may also have to paddle in the hot sun. Early fall is an excellent time to paddle here. Temperatures have moderated and winds are not as frequent as in the spring. Nights can be cold, but the days are usually warm. This pattern can persist until early October, when south-migrating waterfowl are visiting. Winters are not mild in this area, and much of the open water freezes over.

Hazards: Banks Lake's water temperature during the summer is not cold enough to present an unusual hazard. Early spring and late fall water temperatures vary, and it is a good idea during these times to remember that immersion in cold water can be dangerous.

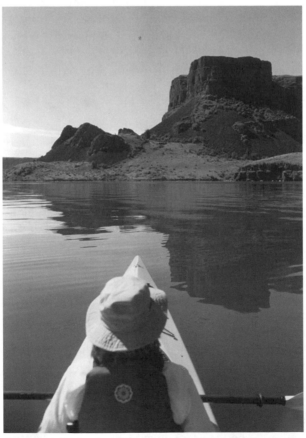

Steamboat Rock, a basaltic promontory that resisted scouring by massive floods, rises above the calm waters of Banks Lake

Located in an area without mountains, Grand Coulee is subject to prevailing winds that sweep across the plateau above. The orientation of Banks Lake within the coulee parallels certain prevailing winds, which can be strong out on the lake. The southern half of the lake has no protecting coves along the west shore, so if a wind comes up, you either weather it, land, or cross the lake (20 minutes paddling) before the wind arrives. This lake is large enough for serious wind waves to form, so keep an eye out for signs of approaching wind.

Mosquitoes can be annoying for short periods in the spring. Take repellent with you, as some of the pests can persist into summer. Remember also that this is snake habitat. Look before you leap ashore, and look over your campsite before relaxing there.

How to Get There

Take I-90 to the town of Moses Lake in central Washington (100 miles west of Spokane). Drive north 47 miles from Moses Lake on Hwy. 17 to Dry Falls Junction at the south end of Banks Lake. Turn right (east) on Hwy. 2 and drive across Dry Falls Dam to Coulee City. Continue east 2 miles through Coulee City to the junction with Hwy. 155. Turn left (north) on 155, and proceed 14 miles to Steamboat Rock State Park.

Area Features, Background, and Tips

Seventeen million years ago lava flowed to the earth's surface near what is now the border of eastern Washington and Oregon. Basaltic lava spread out over the country, filling stream valleys with dams that caused lakes. The mighty Columbia River was forced into its present course as lava flowed northwest. Flow after flow spread out and cooled, stacked like the layers in a cake. For 11 million years this volcanic activity continued, until 63,000 square miles of the Pacific Northwest lay beneath layers, which were in places nearly 2 miles thick. Today, this area is known as the Columbia Plateau. After the lava flows ceased, the plateau was gradually lifted and tilted slightly south by tectonic forces, resulting in a fracturing and stair-stepping of the individual flow layers.

About a million years ago—around the beginning of the Pleistocene Epoch—cooling climatic conditions marked the beginning of the Great Ice Age. Ice sheets formed when more snow fell each year than melted or evaporated. At higher elevations ice sheets became thousands of feet thick, and began moving down slope under the influence of gravity. Pressure from ice to the north kept the glaciers moving, and advancing south into Washington, Idaho, and Montana. The leading edges of the glaciers dammed rivers with ice, creating lakes. One tongue of this glacial sheet reached and blocked the

Columbia River downstream from the present site of Grand Coulee Dam. The blocked water rose in an ever-increasing lake until it finally broke through landforms containing it on the south and, aided by the plateau's south tilt, cut a new channel that rejoined the old one 70-80 miles downstream. This channel was the beginning of the Grand Coulee.

Meanwhile, another glacial tongue had blocked a fork of the Snake River, backing water into what eventually became Lake Missoula in present-day Montana. It covered hundreds of square miles and impounded so much water that it's hard to imagine. At some point Lake Missoula broke through the ice dam, unleashing a flood that for volume may have been unequaled. Tremendous flows rushed across northern Idaho and into eastern Washington, generally channeling along the Columbia River. The flows rushed through Grand Coulee, gouging, tearing, and ripping at soil and fractured basalt layers. Time after time catastrophic floods raced across the region during the ice age. The ice dam blocking the Columbia shunted these floods into the Grand Coulee.

Two major waterfalls formed along the coulee, the larger one 800 feet high. So great was the force of the water that the precipice forming one fall was plucked away, causing a gradual erosion that moved upstream until the fall eventually cut through to the old Columbia River channel near Grand Coulee Dam and disappeared. The layered nature of the basalt also enabled floods to create present-day Dry Falls, another precipice that originated near Soap Lake, and was gradually retreating upstream as the tremendous erosive powers of the torrent yanked chunks of rock from the face of the fall.

Undoubtedly Dry Falls would have eventually retreated until it self-destructed by cutting through into the old Columbia channel, but a warming climate brought about another change. The ice damming the Columbia River melted, allowing that river to return to its former channel. The Grand Coulee was now isolated several hundred feet above the level of the Columbia River. No longer eroded by torrential waters, Dry Falls stands a few miles south of Banks Lake as a reminder to the catastrophic floods. South of Grand Coulee the floods spread wider across the countryside, but much cutting and gouging occurred. Today, this area is referred to as the Channeled Scablands.

When Grand Coulee Dam on the Columbia River was in the planning stages, engineers recognized the potential of a reservoir occupying a portion of the nearby Grand Coulee. Two dams were built in the coulee, North Dam at its mouth and Dry Falls Dam about 28 miles down the coulee. Banks Lake was formed between the two dams. A special power plant was built at Grand Coulee Dam expressly for the purpose of pumping Columbia River water up into the Grand Coulee. The effort to design and construct a project of this magnitude has paid dividends in the form of irrigation water for large desert expanses in central Washington, which today are agriculturally productive.

The most scenic portions of Banks Lake are within a 5-mile radius of Steamboat Rock. Colorful lichens paint the basaltic cliffs, which in places plunge vertically into the water. Just up-lake from Steamboat Rock, the jagged peninsula thrusting south from the east shore is mostly granite, different from the widespread basalt. Magma, molten rock that rose up near but cooled before reaching the earth's surface, formed into granite plutons. The lava covering the granite was stripped away by the floods here, revealing the plutons. It's a pleasant contrast.

In the vicinity of North Dam near Electric City the lake has low-lying shorelines for the first 5 miles down-lake. A levee to elevate Highway 155 over an east-shore arm of Banks Lake created Osborne Bay Lake. The west shore here is indented by several long, narrow inlets. There is a boat-launching facility at Electric City, and another just west of the south end of the causeway over Osborne Bay Lake. There is also a launching ramp on a contorted, narrow peninsula along the east shore just east of Steamboat Rock. A half-mile north of this ramp are two islands, of which the northernmost is Eagle Rock. A wind-warning beacon atop the southernmost, unnamed island flashes admonitions when winds become serious. Narrow channels between

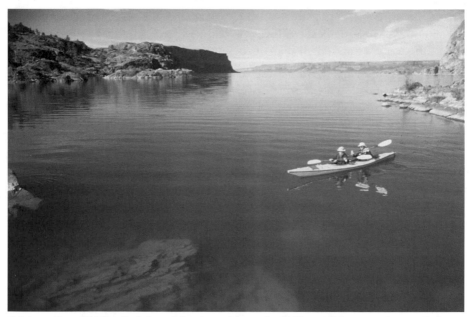

Inlets such as Old Devils Lake are fun to explore and provide excellent campsites nestled along shore

islands in this area are fun to paddle. One mile north of Eagle Rock, near the west shore, is a small granitic islet that might make an intriguing slickrock-type campsite.

Steamboat Rock State Park maintains a boat-in campground, separated from the road-accessible camping areas and located on a gently sloping point. There are 10 spaces with tables, fire rings, and pit toilets. A fee is charged for use of these campsites. They are popular with powerboaters during the summer season. If you don't want company, you may have to look elsewhere.

Within 2 or 3 miles of the north end of Steamboat Rock are several inlets and coves along the southwest shore of the jagged west-shore peninsula. As on any paddling trip, your campsite is where you find a suitable spot. Yet, one idyllic campsite is found at the north end of Old Devils Lake (a cove), and another is in the shallow cove between the two points separating Old Devils Lake and Barker Cove (where there's a large beach and a shade tree). Check also the beach site with a shade tree 0.2 mile inside Old Devils Lake on the west shore. Still other places to check are on the shore directly north of Goose Island.

A camping area with toilets is located at the outflow from Barker Canyon, on the northwest shore. This spot can also be reached by gravel road. Go north 9 miles and then west from the town of Grand Coulee on Hwy. 174, and then turn left (south) on the road marked BARKER CANYON. It is approximately 6 miles to the camping area.

If you don't care to stay at the state park, primitive car camping is possible along the lakeshore at Jones Bay, Million Dollar Mile, and at another launching site 0.5 mile south of Million Dollar Mile. These sites are on the east side of the lake, accessible from Hwy. 155. On the west side is Barker Canyon (mentioned above) and a launching and camping site 1 mile north of Hwy. 2 at Dry Falls Junction. Banks Lake has excellent fishing for warm-water species. Much of the boat traffic on the lake is fishing oriented.

Trip Description

From the main launching ramp at Steamboat Rock State Park, paddle north 0.5 mile and pass through the narrows separating Steamboat from the east-shore peninsula. The boat-in campground is located on the west point at the narrows. Continue 0.6 mile along the east shore of Steamboat Rock to the northernmost point. From here Old Devils Lake lies due north (340° magnetic), 1mile away.

If it's choppy and the prospect of the open crossing to Old Devils Lake is not to your liking, you can paddle 65° east to the closest point of shore. Follow the shoreline north and then east, along a wide, jagged cove. Then, at a small islet just off the point to the north, head north and paddle into Old Devils

Lake. It is 1 mile to the north end of the cove, where there's a small beach beside some rocks just the right height for a camp table. If this site is occupied, remember that there are other sites nearby.

Alternate Trips

You can choose just about any spot on Banks Lake for a destination. Remember that the west shore of the lake is inaccessible to vehicles except at Barker Canyon and via jeep trails at a few points. Exploring the west shore, and finding your own campsite along it, will practically guarantee seclusion. If you paddle this shoreline, keep a watch for petroglyphs on flat basalt surfaces. You can also put your kayak in several of the lakes in Sun Lakes State Park, farther south in the coulee off of Hwy. 17 just south of Coulee City. None of the lakes are large, but each has a distinct character.

Other Area Activities

A day spent sightseeing in the area would be incomplete without a visit to Dry Falls. The visitor center there is rich with interpretive material about formation of the fall, the coulee, and the Channeled Scablands. Lenore Caves, a few miles south of Dry Falls, are worth a visit. Native Americans used them as shelters and for storage. At day's end, consider driving to Grand Coulee Dam and taking in the laser light show there. Each evening during the season, lights are projected onto the dam's concrete surface, accompanied by music, narration, and sound effects. Times for the show vary with the coming of darkness.

Contacts

Steamboat Rock State Park
Reservations: (800) 452-5687

For information on the Grand Coulee Dam light show, and general area information:

Grand Coulee Power Office
PO Box 620
Grand Coulee, WA 99133-0620
(509) 633-9265

It was what some people call a duster, except we were on the water and the waves were raising the bow of our double kayak a couple of feet each time a crest rolled by. There was nothing wrong with our speed, since we were heading north and the wind was from the south. The major complication was an angle with the overtaking waves

that threatened to slew the stern to starboard. Had we been far from shore and the water cold, it would have been white-knuckle time.

But this was Banks Lake; the water temperature was moderate, and we only had a mile to go. So, with some judicious application of rudder and paddle to avoid broaching, we coasted the remainder of the crossing and entered a long, narrow bay. In a few hundred feet the wind waves diminished, and we were paddling normally. Ashore, a great blue heron we hadn't seen decided we were invading its territory and, with a loud squawk, flapped ponderously away. We continued up the bay.

The rocks here were coarse-grained granite, their light gray color contrasting with the dark, lichen-studded cliffs we had left half an hour ago. The decomposition of granite results in coarse sand and, sure enough, we soon saw an inviting beach, which would have made a fine campsite had not our destination been more distant. We paddled along the shore, still pushed somewhat by the tailwind. A pile of rushes—the dwelling of a muskrat—slid by and was soon far astern.

When we reached our intended site, an angler's boat was pulled up on the beach. We drifted for a while, but there was no indication that the anglers were about to leave. We could always return to the first beach, but it might be fun to try finding an alternate location. The bay continued for a half-mile, so we paddled along slowly, evaluating every camping possibility.

We passed huge boulders jutting from the water, defining narrow passages. The head of the bay slipped by the port side, without offering any promising campsite. We followed the shoreline curve around, and began paddling out of the bay against the wind. There was nothing for the first few hundred yards, and then we saw a narrow beach—not more than 8 feet wide—flanked on either side by granite boulders at the water line. As we drew abreast of the beach, it was evident that the sand ran up a few yards, and then turned to green grass on a flat above the watermark. But the beach was too narrow; we couldn't land parallel the shore, as we usually do.

A smaller boulder's rounded surface projecting out of water a yard from shore provided the answer. We pulled the boat alongside, disembarked one at a time onto the boulder, and sloshed through the shallow water to shore. When we pulled the length of the boat onto the beach, the bow reached nearly up to the grass. Our gear was accessible, the boat was protected by the boulder, and our tent would be out of the wind. It was hard to imagine a more intimate site.

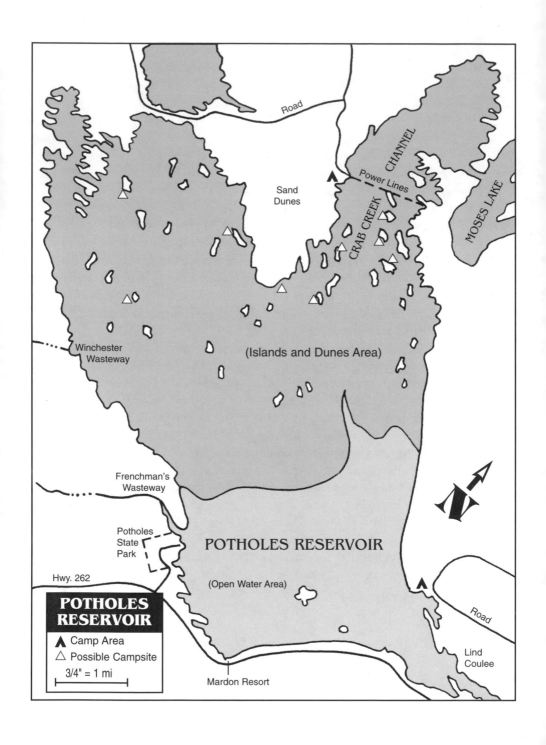

Washington

Chapter 6

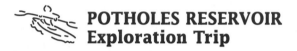 **POTHOLES RESERVOIR**
Exploration Trip

Trip Details

Distance:	11 miles
Time:	5 hours paddling
Rating:	Easy to Moderate
Maps:	USGS 7.5-min: *O'Sullivan Dam*, *Moses Lake South*, *Mae*, and *Royal Camp*

Summary and Highlights

Paddling on Potholes is different; there aren't any nearby mountains. Except for rolling hills at the south end of the reservoir which rise 600 feet above the lake, the region is relatively flat. Navigation is a challenge on this large, island-studded lake where shoreline topography is obscure or lacking. But what a joy to poke around the many willow-shrouded islands, finding different coves and sandy beaches with the varying water level. Campsites abound on the hundreds of islands that were once sand dunes before being partially inundated. So if you have always wanted to find your own private campsite on an island, Potholes is the place!

Because there are so many campsites, and consequently destinations, on Potholes Reservoir, the trip described is just one of many possibilities. It would be nearly impossible to pinpoint each campsite, or to mark them all on a map. So I'll mark a few, but let you to use the skills described at the beginning of this book to find the one you enjoy most. The only developed facilities are those at Potholes State Park and at a half-dozen launching ramps. For this reason, the trip begins and ends at Potholes State Park, an oasis of green in a desert environment with tent and RV camping and lake access.

As you paddle this route, you will experience both the lake's open-water expanses as well as the intricate channels and coves between the sand islands. Pushing through shallow areas, you'll move aside willow wands, which project above the surface but don't pose a barrier to your kayak. And you will see—up close and at water level—the animal life of this desert ecosystem. Besides the myriad birds, beavers are numerous in the reservoir. Paddling here is like being on a wildlife refuge.

When to go: In April there are plenty of ducks and geese, a few swans, and some cranes on the reservoir, remnants of the northward migration. Usually, spring runoff has filled the lake by then. As spring progresses, the numbers of waterfowl decrease as northbound birds leave. Resident birds are active and visible until they begin nesting. From late April on, you will see little of them because they are on the nest. In early summer you may see ducklings and goslings. In the fall, the southbound waterfowl migration begins and large numbers of birds visit the area.

Weather is a primary factor in planning when to go. While spring and fall are pleasant, cold periods can occur anytime. Wind and unsettled weather is most likely in spring. During summer, when temperatures are quite warm, winds often remain calm. Summer heat can be well over 100° by midday, a time when you may prefer to be in camp somewhere under a willow—free to jump into the water when you feel like it. Winters cannot be considered mild.

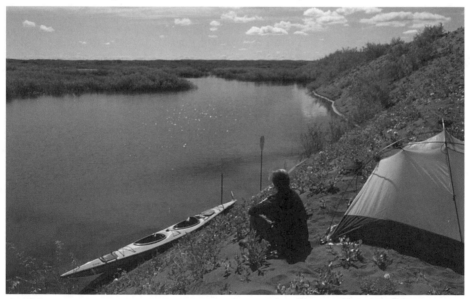

Sand dunes in the northern half of Potholes Reservoir provide scores of secluded campsites at various water levels

Below-freezing temperatures occur often and lakes in the area commonly freeze over.

Hazards: The paddling is easy here, except when wind blows across the open expanses. The moderate rating for this trip is due to the possibility of wind arising. The central part of Potholes is about 9 square miles, plenty of open water to get mighty choppy if a stiff wind comes up. Crossing that expanse east-west, or north-south, is a 3-mile paddle, and the weather can change in the hour it takes you to complete the crossing. It is a good idea to get your paddling done early in the day.

Except in early spring and late fall, and of course during winter, Potholes Reservoir water temperature is moderate. Even though such water temperatures mitigate the hypothermia hazard to some degree, it is still best to keep your kayak with the smooth, slippery side down. Though unlikely, rattlesnakes are quite capable of swimming to islands, so look around before making camp and be observant while walking on the shore. Mosquitoes may be pesky during the spring at Potholes.

How to Get There

Take I-90 (running east-west through central Washington) to Moses Lake (100 miles east of Spokane). From Moses Lake, turn south on Hwy. 17. Drive for 10 miles to the junction with Hwy. 262. Turn right and drive west 10 miles to Potholes State Park, crossing O'Sullivan Dam along the way.

Area Features, Background, and Tips

Potholes Reservoir lies in an area geologically known as the Channeled Scablands. About one million years ago, climatic cooling started the most recent ice age. Huge glaciers formed as snowfall exceeded melt and evaporation, and moved south from Canada into Montana, Idaho, and Washington. One result was to form an ice dam blocking a fork of the Snake River that created a huge lake in Montana called Lake Missoula. By the time the ice dam melted and was breached, hundreds of square miles of this lake drained westward in a matter of days, producing a catastrophic flood that followed the general course of the Columbia River. The flow was diverted south by another ice dam near the present site of Grand Coulee Dam. Near Moses Lake, the flood poured unfettered across the land, scouring much of the surface soil from the region and leaving only hard, resistant basalt bedrock and outcroppings. Potholes Reservoir lies in an area scoured out by these floods.

In the Columbia National Wildlife Refuge just south of Potholes Reservoir, hundreds of pothole lakes occupy depressions torn and scoured out by the flood. You can stand at any of several roadside viewpoints and see graphic evidence in the landscape: channels where softer rocks and soil were torn away, towered over by basaltic cliffs and mesas where the water force met its match in hard, resistant rock. (More details on the Lake Missoula floods can be found in Chapter 5.)

Since the time of the floods, the Potholes Reservoir basin has been recovering ever so slowly by soil deposition from gentler runoff and, in some areas, soil particles borne by the wind. Sand dunes formed in the area later flooded by Potholes Reservoir, and extend more than 20 miles west. These dunes form most of the islands in the northern portion of the reservoir.

When the Bureau of Reclamation constructed O'Sullivan Dam across Crab Creek just downstream from its confluence with Lind Coulee, the result was Potholes Reservoir, part of an irrigation project benefiting agriculture in the area. It is basically a shallow impoundment, with depths of less than 100 feet over 95% of the surface area. The Washington State Parks, the state fish and wildlife department, and the Columbia National Wildlife Refuge have all added launching and camping improvements in the area. It is possible to launch a boat at 10 different sites on the reservoir, two sites on Lind Coulee, and half a dozen sites on the pothole lakes dotting the area to the south.

Camping in established, though primitive, sites outside the state park is possible at two gravel launch areas at the north end of the reservoir, at the fish and wildlife launch ramp on Lind Coulee near the east end of the dam, and at several other locations. In addition, camping is permitted at a dozen or so places on fish and wildlife lands adjacent to the Columbia Wildlife Refuge. All of these are within 15 miles of Potholes Reservoir.

Potholes Reservoir is about 10 miles long north and south, and branches into two distinct arms in the northern half. The west arm is 3 miles wide, while the east arm is about half that. The north two thirds of the lake averages only about 15 feet in depth, with the old creek channels deeper in some areas. This north section of the lake is a maze of sand-dune islands that constantly change with varying water level. Willows grow profusely on the islands, mostly at and below the watermark. Even when the lake is full it's common to see willows growing up through the water in the shallower areas.

But many of the dunes rise high enough above the water that their sandy tops are free of vegetation. When such a dune also has a sandy beach, it's a good candidate for a campsite. In general, the west sides of dune islands slope gently and are likely to be covered with willows. The east sides tend to be more abrupt in slope, and generally offer the best landing places. Hundreds of such spots dot the northern reaches of Potholes Reservoir when the lake is full; countless more become feasible campsites as the water level drops. Besides island locations, many shoreline stretches can be considered for campsites.

A word of caution about island camping at Potholes. Vast areas of the lake can be explored to find just the right campsite. But once you've found it, be cautious about paddling away until you're ready to move on. Because much of the area is a confusing maze with few recognizable landmarks, it may be difficult to return to any given spot. You might paddle a mile or so from your camp and have to spend hours of trial and error searching to return. One solution is to place a flag on a pole at the highest point on your island, so it can be seen from afar. Another is to use GPS; finding your way back to camp is a snap if you are proficient with the instrument.

Landmarks are conspicuously absent in this region, making a compass essential. The exception are hills at the reservoir's south end, which rise 600 feet above the 1,046' full-pool level of the lake, offering visual reference. In addition, the hillside south of Potholes State Park is the site of a small housing development. If islands and willows don't block your view, you can spot this developed area and the tall, green poplars at the state park. But the rest of the shore is mostly featureless, especially from kayak level.

Fishing is excellent in Potholes Reservoir. Species commonly fished for are large- and smallmouth bass, walleye, and catfish. There are trout in many of the pothole lakes south of the reservoir.

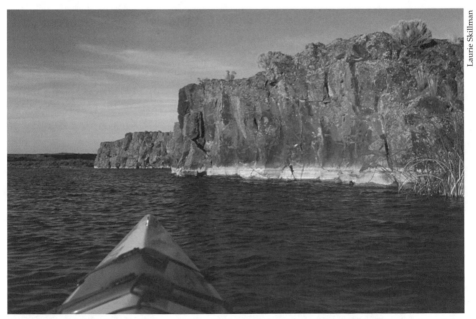

Laurie Skillman

Seclusion, lichen-splayed cliffs, and abundant bird life are benefits of a day trip on Hutchinson & Shiner lakes

A map of underwater contours is helpful when navigating Potholes Reservoir. Marketed by Fish'n'Map Company, the map is a reasonable attempt to locate underwater contours using aerial photos of the lake at various water levels. It may be purchased locally at Mardon Resort (see Contacts) or obtained by calling (303) 421-5994.

Trip Description

From the launching ramp at Potholes State Park, paddle 345° North 4 miles to the main underwater channel of Crab Creek. At this point, the southern tip of the peninsula dividing the two northern arms of Potholes Reservoir lies 1 mile off your port beam bearing 270° West, although you may not be able to differentiate between the peninsula and intervening islands. At full-pool water level, you will have passed near two tiny islets at the 3-mile mark, and you will also notice a confusing sprinkling of islets northwest. These willow-clad dune islets are practically indistinguishable from the shoreline. However, the true western shore of Potholes Reservoir lies more than 3 miles due west, 2 miles beyond the peninsula tip. (If the reservoir water level is down 15 feet or so, you will probably not be able to paddle the direct-line course mentioned above because of shallows and islands. In this event, paddle on a course of 15° for 3 miles to the Crab Creek channel; then turn to port and paddle a course of 310° for 2 miles, following the channel.)

At the 4-mile mark of your paddle (if you paddled 345° at full pool), you should be able to discern the main underwater channel of Crab Creek as it winds through islands from the north. (Two miles north up the channel are a set of power lines, which cross the east arm in a generally east-west direction, making a good landmark. There is a gravel launching ramp here, and people often camp on shore in RVs.) At the 4-mile mark you should be very near two tiny islets, if you stayed on course. One-half mile northwest at 300° is a line of half a dozen, sizable poplar trees. These trees are on an island that is nearly one third of a mile long, and has some nice sandy beaches near the trees on its south tip. Camp here, and you not only have shade but an excellent view south out over the lake.

If the island camp does not suit you, or if it's in use, there are several more sizable islands lying in shallow water directly northwest. These islands become part of the mainland when the water level drops 5 feet or more from full-pool level. In this event, there are some desirable secluded sites on islands lying 30° East of the poplar trees, 0.6 mile distant. Poke among these sandy isles until you find just the right spot. A nice feature here is that some of the islets rise 20 feet or more above the water, providing a better view. In conclusion, water levels and conditions will determine where you camp. The advantage is having so many choices. To return to Potholes State Park, retrace your course.

Additional Trips

While there is plenty of exploring to be done in the east arm of Potholes Reservoir, the west arm is three times as expansive. Instead of having one main channel like Crab Creek, the west arm has two separate channels, which, however, are shallower, less distinct, and harder to follow. Though the west arm poses a much more difficult-to-navigate maze, it also has some nifty, potential campsites and plenty of places to explore. Paddling there does become very challenging if the water level is less than 15 feet of full pool. Winchester Wasteway is a canal system that returns irrigation water to the reservoir. It is located on the west shore, about midway between the north and south ends of the lake.

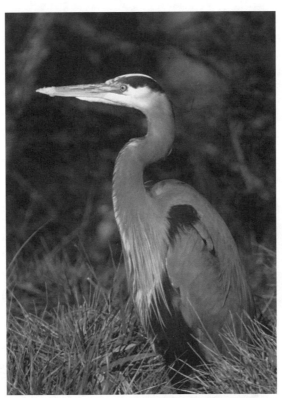

Great blue herons are quite wary in the wild, and your spotting one means that the area has not recently been disturbed by humans

Another interesting paddle is to explore Lind Coulee from the launching ramp at the east end of O'Sullivan Dam. The coulee averages a quarter mile wide, and can be paddled east for about 5 miles, making a nice day trip. Since the coulee lies below the surrounding desert and agricultural land, views from the water level are limited. Depending upon wind direction, paddling the coulee is a good alternative if winds on the main reservoir exceed your comfort zone.

Not to be overlooked are the various lakes in the Columbia National Wildlife Refuge. Access by road is provided to many of these lakes, and all are scenic in their own way. A notable and pleasant day paddle is the 4-mile round trip around the shores of Hutchinson and Shiner lakes, which are narrow lakes connected by a shallow arm. Regulations prohibiting motors assure peace and quiet on these lakes. Be sure to check the regulations and closures in effect before paddling in the refuge. There are geological observation points and interpretive displays at various locations here. Contact the wildlife refuge for more information.

Contacts

Columbia National Wildlife Refuge
PO Drawer F
Othello, WA 99344
(509) 488-2668

Potholes State Park
Northwest Reservations: (800) 452-5687

Mardon Resort
8198 Highway 262 E
Othello, WA 99344
(509) 346-2651

We spotted the rounded, bald dune of dark gray sand from half a mile away, rising 20 feet higher than anything near it. From this distance it seemed to have campsite written all over it; we would have to check it out. The question was how to get there. The channel we were following ran at a right angle to the way we wanted to go. Between us and the dune were who-knows-how-many lesser ones and a labyrinth of channels, all disguised by willows on the shore and willow patches poking here and there above the water. With our map no help, trial and error was the only way.

We were in luck, for a few hundred feet along the channel a shallow waterway led closer to the tall dune. With only inches to spare, we scooted through in our kayak. This channel seemed to lead only slightly closer, until we were able to angle around a large patch of willows and approach the tall dune. We had paddled a mile and a half to cover less than half a mile.

But the spot was worth it. The shallow waterway we had traversed practically guaranteed privacy in the small, secluded cove upon which the steep, sandy beach fronted. No powerboats would intrude here. A few yards inland from the beach was an elevated bench for our tent. It was one of those places that abound in aesthetics: privacy, view, level site, shelter, and our boat below only 30 feet away. Yet the most striking feature was the wildflowers. Hundreds of them practically carpeted the bench. With effort we found a spot to erect the tent without crushing flowers.

After setting up camp, we trudged up to the summit of our dune. From the top we could easily orient ourselves to the rest of the lake. Some eight miles south the ridge of hills near the state park was visible. Below—in our tiny bay—the smooth surface was marred only by a couple of coots puttering about in the willows. We descended the dune's steep east slope, starting minor sand avalanches with each step.

The spring sunshine's warmth was sufficient that we were soon refreshing in the cool water. Afterwards, we dug out canvas backrests and paperbacks and went over to a willow's shade. I was preoccupied with the book until the loud trill of a red-winged blackbird above entered my consciousness. The bay was glassy; the blackbird sang on. This must be what it's all about.

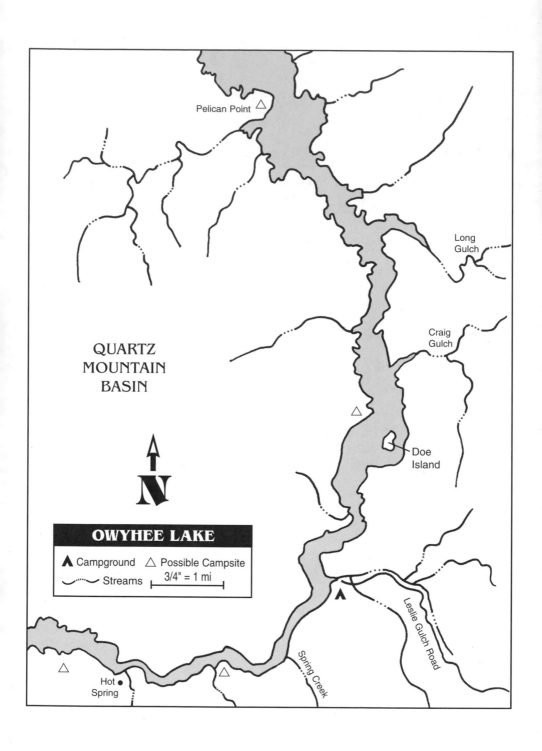

Oregon

Chapter 7

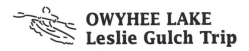 **OWYHEE LAKE
Leslie Gulch Trip**

Trip Details	
Distance:	15 miles
Time:	6 hours paddling
Rating:	Easy
Maps:	USGS 7.5-min: *Rooster Comb, Pelican Point, Diamond Butte,* and *The Elbow*

Summary and Highlights

This trip is reminiscent of paddling in the spectacular red-rock country of the Southwest. Bighorn sheep come down to water, eagles soar, and chukar partridge call from the sagebrush. The quiet feeling of a vast, remote desert landscape is pervasive. This landscape seems strangely out of place because Lake Owyhee is in southeastern Oregon, one of the most lightly populated areas in the U.S. The lake (actually a reservoir) is 36 miles in length and averages less than a mile wide. Southern stretches are held between spectacular cliffs and steep shorelines of red, orange, and yellow rock. Shades of the Colorado Plateau! What is all this doing here?

The natural features make paddling here interesting. The lake's narrow configuration and its geographical location help minimize wind patterns that build uncomfortable wind waves. The sinuous oxbow bends of the reservoir over much of its length also provide ample sheltered water and minimize fetch.

Shoreline camping is allowed at Owyhee, and there are adequate sites where camping is both feasible and enjoyable. A few of these possible sites even have shade trees. Unlike some impoundments that receive intensive recreational usage, you won't have any competition from houseboats for the same campsite. And in the upper lake, where most of the boating is related to the excellent fishing, you will have your pick of shoreline sites. While the hot spring is a popular spot, usage is not so continuous that you won't have a turn. Warm water from the spring is piped out to a showering location, a real treat in this area being considered for wilderness status. You may spot bighorn sheep, as there are nearly 200 in Leslie Gulch and the surrounding area. These animals have increased from an initial reintroduction of 17 animals in 1965. Mule deer are present in the area, and a few Rocky Mountain elk are found here.

But your first feeling of awe when entering the area via Leslie Gulch will come from the honeycombed towers and cliffs, which you see right from the road. Many are hundreds of feet high, presenting rugged, eroded surfaces and photogenic outlines. Turn and look up-canyon in the afternoon, and the golden light of sunset fans the area as if afire. Then, when you spot this narrow corridor of lake nestled in the canyon bottom, holding out the promise of paddling among these colorful cliffs, you will want to get your boat in the water right away. If the relatively short trip detailed here is not enough for you, simply continue down-lake as far as you want. Some tips on camping

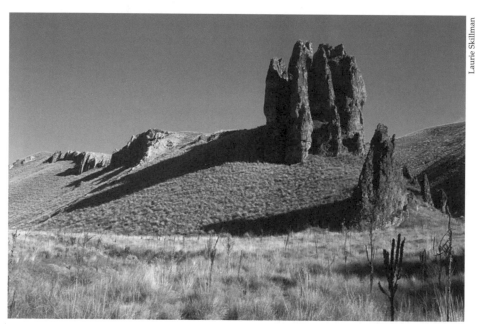

Laurie Skillman

Spires of vocanic tuff add allure to paddling on Owyhee Lake

areas and spots of interest in the rest of the lake are detailed later in this chapter.

When to go: Because winters are cold in this high-desert environment, the best paddling is May through October. If spring is late or fall early, access to Leslie Gulch may be impaired by snow or mud. Check with administrative agencies before traveling at either end of the season. Spring days are cool, with occasional storms passing through but rarely lasting long. The lake can be full in the spring, with water levels dropping later in the season. Summer temperatures can be on the hot side—over 100°—so if you go during this season, be prepared to carry a sunshade to use in camp. As in all warm, dry climates, be sure to drink enough water. Thunderstorms are possible in late spring and during the summer. Fall days can be warm, with nights increasingly chilly as the season progresses.

Hazards: While Owyhee is not noted for severe wind patterns, it is a large body of water and winds are possible. If severe wind waves do occur, it is usually only a short paddle to a sheltered spot or a landing place. Rapidly changing weather can also affect road and driving conditions on the way into Leslie Gulch. There are no services available; the closest are in Homedale and Jordan Valley.

When ashore, remember that rattlesnakes are found here. Use caution when walking in likely areas.

You may want to carry all of your drinking water for your trip on Owyhee. You will need to carry all your water for camping at Leslie Gulch also. While you can treat the lake water, it may be unappetizing at various times of the year due to sedimentation or algae bloom.

How to Get There

From Ontario, Oregon, near the Oregon-Idaho border, drive 5 miles southeast on I-84 into Idaho to the intersection with Hwy. 95. Turn right (south) on Hwy. 95 and drive 26 miles to Homedale. Turn right (west) on Hwy. 19 at Homedale, and proceed 7 miles to the junction with Hwy. 201. Turn left (south) on gravel-surfaced 201 and go approximately 25 miles through the Succor Creek State Recreation Area to the signed intersection with a gravel road heading west (right) to Leslie Gulch. Turn right and go approximately 15 miles to the camping and launching area.

Area Features, Background, and Tips

While most of the landscape of southeastern Oregon was formed primarily by faulting rather than by erosion, the picturesque towers in Leslie Gulch and elsewhere in the Owyhee Canyon are an exception. The other-worldly formations of Leslie Gulch are formed of volcanic tuff, which is ash cemented into a layer with structural strength but soft enough to erode and weather. These 15-million-year-old formations are composed of air-fall ash that erupted from a local volcano in a series of explosions. Ash falling back into the volcano's caldera formed a gaseous deposit of small rocks and ash up to 1,000 feet thick. This is the layer, solidified, from which the striking formations have been carved. The tuff contains minerals, the source of the reds and oranges that so quickly catch the eye.

Generally, the landforms of the region were created by faulting, the movement of blocks of crust upward to form scarps or ridges, or downward to form valleys. Since the area is semiarid, there is not enough water to carry away the products of erosion; scourings from higher areas move only as far as lower-lying spots in the locality. While spring floods on the Owyhee River are capable of moving quantities of material, most sediments weathered or eroded from higher slopes are still present in the valleys. Surface and underlying rocks are volcanic in origin.

Leslie Gulch is representative of the more scenic areas along the Owyhee, but it is uncommon to the extent it was designated an Area of Critical Environmental Concern in 1983, to protect the area's wilderness from deterioration until Congress decides whether to grant it formal "Wilderness" status. Specific clays and volcanic-derived soils support rare native plants. Several other large tracts of land in the general area are presently undergoing study as prospective wilderness areas.

Native American peoples hunted and gathered in the area for 5,000 years or more. A few, isolated petroglyph sites in the canyon now lie beneath the lake. Usage by early inhabitants was probably intermittent, depending upon fish in the river and availability of seasonal, edible plants and nuts. Game species such as deer and waterfowl were present but not unusually abundant. The land then was much as you see it today, starkly beautiful, but not overly hospitable. The climate was probably wetter than it is today.

Owyhee Lake is a reservoir, created on the Owyhee River by Owyhee Dam, a hydroelectric project of the U.S. Bureau of Reclamation. While most of the shoreline is Bureau of Reclamation land, land farther from the water is administered by the Bureau of Land Management. A few areas of the shore are privately owned. Camping is allowed along the shoreline on the public land.

The terrain is quite rugged. Covered as it is with sage and other brush as well as native grasses, it's easy to imagine that you are an early explorer as you paddle slowly by. The elevation is moderate, with the plateau above the Owyhee drainage averaging about 3,500 feet. Mule deer are the most numerous large animal you are likely to see. A few elk winter in the area, but don't expect to see them.

More visible in the Leslie Gulch area are the bighorn sheep. These animals are the result of a dedicated reintroduction program in Oregon, which is a refreshing success story. As a result of this effort, bighorn sheep again occupy their historic ranges in many areas not only in Oregon, but in neighboring states as well. The Leslie Gulch area is ideal sheep habitat, for not only are the necessary food plants present, the topography provides steep slopes and cliffs that sheep need to escape predators. At present, these predators are coyotes and an occasional cougar.

Many raptor nesting sites are found in cliffs along the lake, especially in the more rugged terrain of the upper (southern) portions. Eagles—both golden and bald—can be found here. Osprey can often be observed fishing successfully in the lake waters. California quail inhabit the more open ground ashore, while chukar partridge are frequently seen, usually while coming

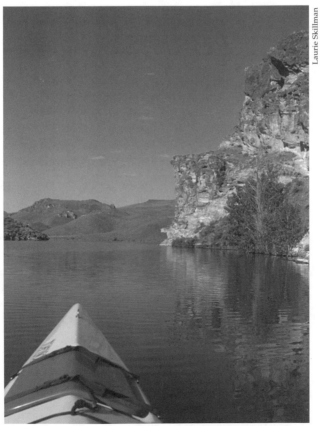

Exploring this inlet near Leslie Gulch reveals shoreline cottonwood trees

down to water from steep, rocky slopes. Keep watch while paddling or resting, and you will see other birds and possibly a coyote or bobcat.

The narrow configuration of Owyhee Lake makes it an enjoyable place to paddle. Even if you decide to cross from one side to the other, such crossings are rarely more than a half mile (requiring about 10 minutes of paddling time). You can do a lot of exploring here because of the substantial length of the lake. There are plenty of coves and water-filled gulches to pique your interest, too.

The north (downstream) end of the lake has more private ownership. Many people have built cabins along the lakeshore, especially along the west shore just north of the lake's midpoint. Reminiscent of older styles, most of these places are modest shelters for a few days respite on a remote lake. One bay in particular with over a half mile of frontage hosts a dozen or more such cabins. This level of development fits in with the landscape much better than would larger, overbuilt vacation homes.

The presence of cabins does not particularly detract from the remote paddling experience. Except for a few concentrations, such structures are well scattered. The northern portions of the lake—with many haul-out spots and possible campsites—have a gentler topography than around Leslie Gulch. On the west shore just 0.5 mile south of the Dry Creek Arm is a possible site with a beach and shade trees. The 2.5-mile-long Dry Creek Arm is an interesting paddling area with only a few cabins near its western end.

At Pelican Point, on the west shore about 8 miles north of Leslie Gulch, is a landing strip with an unimproved dirt runway. Occasionally, pilots of private planes gain access via this strip to camp along the lakeshore. West and up-lake from Leslie Gulch just 3.8 miles by water, on the south shore, is a hot spring. The flow is channeled through a pipe, which forms a makeshift, open-air shower. While the water temperature is comfortable for bathing, don't use soap here or near any natural water feature to safeguard the delicate ecology. Even at full pool—when some reservoirs can be stingy with possible campsites—Owyhee holds out a great spot to tempt you every couple of miles. Such conditions are dear to the hearts of adventure kayakers. Of course, when the water level drops, site possibilities increase as shallow points and cove beaches are uncovered.

The Leslie Gulch launching area is reached by a road that is passable to ordinary vehicles. In the winter, the access road is often blocked by snow or impossibly muddy. While Owyhee State Park, at the north end of the lake near the dam, is reached by a paved road, all other lake access points require a 4WD vehicle. To determine conditions at any specific time, contact the BLM office in Vale.

The camping area at Leslie Gulch consists of nothing more than a flat area and two pit toilets. Without available drinking water, there are no facilities here other than the well-designed launching ramp. Because of its lack of amenities, Leslie Gulch is used by those willing to forego some conveniences in exchange for access to a remote section of the lake and camping in view of jagged, eroded towers and cliffs. It is a favored spot for anglers after game fish. Owyhee Lake contains an abundance of carp. Most of the fish you see will be these bronze-sided scavengers. When you spot an osprey swooping down and picking up a fish in its talons, the chances are that the fish is a carp. Anglers aren't after carp; they are pursuing bass or other game fish.

For various reasons at different seasons, the water in Owyhee Lake may not be as clear as you would like it to be. When water temperatures increase in the middle of summer, algae blooms may affect the water quality for drink-

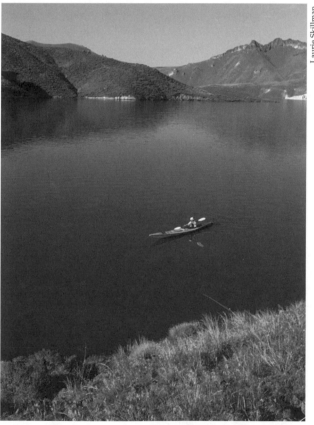

Laurie Skillman

The east end of Owyhee's Doe Island offers an intriguing campsite, but the wildflower-studded peninsula is very fragile

ing purposes. Or spring runoff may muddy the water. It is still safe to drink if you treat or boil it, but it may not be clear or without a taste or odor. If this is objectionable to you, it is best to carry all the water you will need for your trip.

Photography is particularly inspired in the Leslie Gulch area. By determining that a specific cliff or formation faces east or west, and will receive either the low light of sunrise or the sun's rays just before sunset, you can make your photo during these times of golden light. The natural color of the light hitting the escarpments at low angles enhances the inherent colors of the rock, and guarantees a photo to be treasured. In the spring and fall, taking photos on the water while facing north lends the water a deeper blue. This phenomenon causes even slightly muddy water to appear blue in the photo. The north sky has a darker blue than the south in all seasons.

Trip Description

From the Leslie Gulch launch area, paddle north along the east shore. Within 1 mile, you will see some of the vertical cliffs that make this section an inspiring paddle. Enjoy paddling along the base of these ramparts, which are in the shade before noon. At mile 2, you round a point on your right, beyond which the lake stretches to a mile wide. A half mile ahead near the east shore is 400-yard-long Doe Island. The slight peninsula and ridge on the east side of this island offers a tempting camping site. However, if you stay here, be careful not to damage the delicate plants and shrubs on the island. Paintbrush and lupine are abundant, as is purple sage. More than a dozen less common species bloom here at various times. (North of Doe Island 0.5 mile on the west shore, two trees right at the high water line mark a good spot for a camp.)

From Doe Island continue north 1 mile to the entrance of Craig Gulch (3.5 miles from launch). The opening from the east results in a 0.3-mile-long inlet, which is fun to explore. Continue north 0.5 mile from Craig Gulch to a narrows, where points of land projecting from both shores constrict the lake to less than 0.2 mile wide. Several tiny inlets along the west shore are interesting to explore in this section.

North of the constricting points 1.5 miles, Long Gulch enters from the east, forming another interesting inlet more than 0.5 mile in length. The stretch north of Long Gulch is less than 0.5 mile wide, and remains so for over a mile. There are interesting coves here, especially along the east shore. On the northeast shore a cabin, on a point where the lake widens, is the southernmost of a scattering of summer cottages built along the lake's northern shores.

One mile northwest of this cabin, across the lake on the west shore, is easily recognizable Pelican Point. You may see the windsock that tells wind direction to the occasional pilot landing on the unimproved dirt strip here.

There are several campsites under trees along the west shore of the lake, a few hundred yards south of the point (7.5 miles from launch). Retrace the route paddled to return to Leslie Gulch.

Additional Trips

To extend your trip on Owyhee, you can spend a day paddling up-lake (west) from Leslie Gulch. The lake in this section averages only 0.25 mile wide. The hot spring is 3.5 miles west of Leslie Gulch on the south shore. If the lake is at full pool, you can paddle approximately 8 miles west from Leslie Gulch before encountering the shallows and current of incoming Owyhee River. A round trip to the river inflow would make a full day for most paddlers.

To expand the scope of your trip, consider exploring the lake *north* of Pelican Point. On the east shore 2.5 miles north of the point is a shallow bay known as Bensley Flat; there are groves of trees and many camping areas on Bureau of Reclamation land here. On the west shore 0.5 mile north of the flat, a 0.6-mile-long peninsula juts east into the lake, creating a narrow inlet to the north (10.5 miles from Leslie Gulch). Cabins dot the shore every mile or so in this section.

On the west shore 15 miles north of Leslie Gulch is a feature called "The Elbow." This is an old oxbow bend in the river, and flooding has turned the elevated strip of land in the middle of the bend into an island. It is an interesting place; when we visited a mule deer doe had just swum from the mainland to the island to fawn, perhaps because the island offers refuge from coyotes.

Dry Creek Arm, 2.5 miles north of The Elbow, extends west for 2.5 miles and is one of a few areas of the lake accessible via 4WD roads. The 6-mile section up-lake from Dry Creek to Lake Owyhee State Park offers rugged shorelines and colorful outcroppings, and is free of development. Owyhee Dam is 2 miles north of the park. Launching at this end of the lake is at the state park, reached by paved road from the north. The 3 miles of road from the dam to the park—although paved—is not for the fainthearted.

Contacts

Bureau of Land Management
100 Oregon Street
Vale, OR 97918
(541) 473-3144

Lake Owyhee State Park
(541) 339-2331

We had just paddled out of shadow into sunlight, which now reflected from the lightly riffled water. Being left behind was that incredible cliff, its surface of earth-tone yellows and oranges towering far above the water. Now the sun made its warmth felt on this morning in Owyhee country. In the shade of the cliff we had paddled briskly; now we slowed to a speed that was comfortable in the hot sun.

Along the shore somewhere ahead, a chukar called. Soon we spotted a flock of the partridges, running up the steep bank. A dozen yards away, one bird jumped up on a boulder and posed, watching us. Then it darted away, disappearing mysteriously as had the rest of the flock. We dug out binoculars, but the birds were nowhere in sight.

While we were glassing, a prairie falcon swept into view. Rapid wingbeats carried the raptor directly toward a cliff some distance from the water. Just as it seemed that the gray missile must be smashed against the rock, there was a sudden spreading of wings, and the bird settled onto a nest. The aerie was in a tiny alcove in the vertical face. We could understand the nest location; it was a place no land predator could reach.

The kayak was drifting because we hadn't paddled while watching the bird. We were content to let the drift continue for a while. We drank from our water bottles as a slight breeze carried the boat close to shore. Any disturbance our paddling had caused was long passed; we felt like part of the landscape. We could hear the sound of insects ashore, and the tinkling of riffles against rocks. We were at peace and enjoying it, when suddenly the water close to shore erupted as if stirred by a giant egg-beater. It took us a few seconds to recover from the surprise; it was only a school of carp spawning. As we watched, their golden-brown bodies darted down and away.

Paddling lazily now, we looked ahead to where a small cottonwood graced the shore at the water line. There seemed to be a narrow beach. A few minutes later and we were certain; it would be our campsite. There was no need to hurry—the site wasn't going anywhere—so we continued ghosting along shore. We were nearly beyond the east-facing slope slipping behind our boat when we saw the flowers. A solitary bush of purple sage, ablaze in the color of royalty, outshone other vegetation. As if sprinkled from a salt shaker, a mix of crimson paintbrush and blue lupine dotted the slope around the sage. Yes, this would be a good camp.

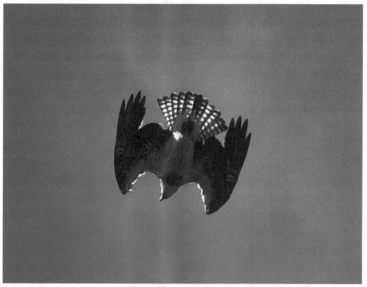

Osprey stooping toward a fish spotted in the water

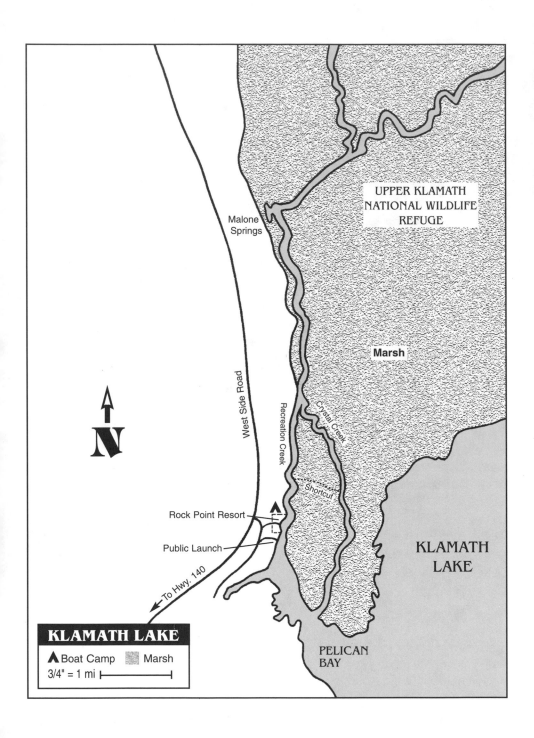

UPPER KLAMATH
NATIONAL WILDLIFE
REFUGE

Malone
Springs

Marsh

West Side Road

Recreation Creek

Crystal Creek

Shortcut

Rock Point Resort

Public Launch

To Hwy. 140

KLAMATH
LAKE

PELICAN
BAY

KLAMATH LAKE

▲ Boat Camp   ▨ Marsh

3/4" = 1 mi ├──────────┤

Oregon

Chapter 8

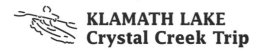

KLAMATH LAKE
Crystal Creek Trip

Trip Details	
Distance:	7-mile day trip
Time:	4 hours paddling
Rating:	Easy
Maps:	USGS 7.5-min: *Crystal Spring*, *Pelican Bay*, and *Agency Lake*

Summary and Highlights

Two things make this trip a joy: very protected water, and the amount of wildlife that can be seen. Less experienced kayakers will appreciate the many miles of narrow, meandering creek channel without noticeable current. More gung-ho paddlers will enjoy taking it easy and reveling in the sights and sounds of the area. The springs that form Crystal Creek flow from the ground at or near lake level, yet generate enough current to open a passageway through the bullrushes, cattails, and pond lilies of the marsh. This freshwater marsh is so important as bird habitat that it has been set aside as the Upper Klamath National Wildlife Refuge. The narrow, open waterways meandering through the heart of the refuge are unusual and offer a unique trip, free from the threat of rough water. Cooperation between the Winema National Forest and the U.S Fish and Wildlife Service has resulted in opening this route, called the Upper Klamath Canoe Trail.

The Upper Klamath National Wildlife Refuge provides nesting habitat for 170 different species of birds. More than 250 species have been seen here. Accordingly, it is a paradise for observing birds from your kayak. Dozens of common species such as mallards, teal, pintails, Canada geese, redwing blackbirds, yellow-headed blackbirds, marsh wrens, and western grebes are seen frequently. There is a good chance of seeing more unique birds like red-necked grebes, sandhill cranes, wood ducks, white pelicans, least bitterns, ospreys, and bald eagles. By paddling slowly or drifting, you can move through the marsh with a minimum of disturbance, one of the enviable abilities of sleek, low-to-the-water, paddle craft.

Those huge mounds of peeled sticks and logs you see occasionally are beaver lodges. These aquatic rodents are sometimes seen in the late evening as they begin their nocturnal activity. But don't be too surprised if a beaver announces its presence with a loud tail slap at any time of the day. You probably won't be looking in that direction and, when you turn your head, all that remains will be rings spreading on the surface. Muskrats are active during daylight hours; that V-shaped wake in the water, formed by eyes and nose above the surface, is a muskrat en route to somewhere. The animals will paddle across the channel in front of you or will swim along the shore. Seen less frequently are the river otters—singly or in groups—diving as they move along the creek channel in search of food. You may also spot mule deer along the wooded portions of the shore.

This trip is designed as a day trip in the marsh and refuge, protected from the open portion of Klamath Lake by dense aquatic vegetation. Klamath Lake is 17 miles long and averages 5 miles in width. Joined to Klamath Lake by a narrow waterway at the north end is 8-mile-long Agency Lake. There is no shortage of water for those who want to paddle longer distances. Two overnight paddles are suggested at the end of this chapter.

When to go: Late spring, summer, and early fall are the best times to schedule a paddle here. Klamath Lake freezes in the winter. The lake is usually ice-

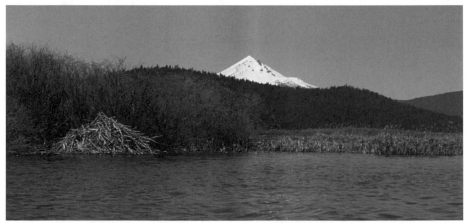

A beaver lodge—common along Klamath Lake shore—with Mt. McLoughlin in the distance

free sometime in early March. Freeze-up can occur in the fall anytime after mid-November. Prior to June, the rushes and cattails are brown and matted down from heavy winter snows. Birds that nest here are courting. The marsh comes alive with new, green growth in late spring and early summer, as tules and rushes rejuvenate for the season. Later in the summer, pond lilies achieve their growth, dotting patches on the surface with bright yellow blossoms. Summer brings warm-to-hot days with cool nights.

Frost will brown the plants by early October, but aspens and cottonwoods will shimmer in the gold of fall. Often fall nights are cold but days are mild and bright. The first waves of migrating waterfowl arrive at the marsh then, adding their numbers to those that have summered here. The highest concentrations are present in November just before the lake freezes. Paddling this route in late fall requires dedication to withstand the chilly temperatures, but can be very rewarding to the bird enthusiast.

Hazards: The water in Klamath Lake comes from springs and spring-fed rivers, as well as spring snowmelt, all very cold. So water temperatures can be low in the channels you will paddle on this trip, while out in the open lake sun may have warmed the surface layers. Consider that the water will be colder than you would care to swim in, and keep your boat upright.

While this trip is in protected waters where wind waves are usually quite small, the alternate trips described at the end of this chapter are in the main lake where wind can be a hazard. Watch for wind if you venture out onto the main lake. There are few coves for shelter; if wind waves occur that are beyond your comfort level, head for shore. This is not always easy to do, as shore can be a solid green wall of impenetrable bullrushes, with adjoining water several feet deep.

Mosquitoes can be numerous in late spring and during the summer. These pests are somewhat lessened when you are out on the water, but camp is another matter. Take a good repellent.

How to Get There

From the junction of Hwy. 97 and Hwy. 140 at the south end of Klamath Falls, turn northwest onto Hwy. 140. Drive 26 miles on 140 to the junction with the West Side Road (the only paved, two-lane highway heading north off 140). Turn right (north) onto the West Side Road and drive approximately 2 miles to the sign ROCKY POINT RESORT AND MARINA. Turn right and drive 0.2 mile to the marina. From I-5 at Medford, drive east 6 miles on Hwy. 62 to the junction with Hwy. 140. Turn right (east) on Hwy. 140 and proceed 47 miles to the junction with the West Side Rd. Turn left (north) and proceed as above.

Area Features, Background, and Tips

The most visible features around Klamath Lake are the volcanos. Just 30 miles north is Crater Lake, which was formed when Mount Mazama exploded 6,700 years ago and rained dozens of cubic miles of ash over Oregon and Northern California. Sixty miles south is Mount Shasta, at 14,162 feet the second highest Cascade volcano in the coterminous United States. Shasta is active with frequently occurring tremors, and summiteers experience the bubbling, sulfurous hot spring near the top. Fifteen miles west of Klamath Lake, Mount McLoughlin rises to 9,495 feet in a classic volcanic cone. This composite volcano probably started building about 1 million years ago, about the same time that Mount Mazama was raising its massive bulk. Closer still is Brown Mountain; cross-country skiers sometimes notice a warm area near the summit where winter snows melt quickly on the ground. Brown Mountain spewed out an extensive lava flow about 17,000 years ago. Pelican Butte, over 8,000 feet high, is omnipresent 4 miles to the west while paddling this trip, its jagged north face the victim of glacial disfiguring.

Don't worry, though. Seismologists tell us that this section of the Cascade Mountains is not scheduled for an eruption anytime soon. These are young mountains as major ranges go. Uplifting began only about five million years ago. Then came the volcanos, which endured the ice age that ended around 12,000 years ago. Glacial ice scoured the highest mountains, resulting in jagged peaks and steep slopes.

The broad valley south of Klamath Lake is mostly agricultural today, and was formed from ash and sediments washed down from the Cascades. Much of the present valley is old lake bottom, some of it reclaimed by draining relic lakes, which were remnants of prehistoric lakes in the valley bottom. Tule Lake and Lower Klamath Lake, 40 miles south of Klamath Lake, are such relics.

The Cascade Mountains, which border the Upper Klamath Lake National Wildlife Refuge, are heavily timbered in this region. Part of the route follows a timbered shoreline, showcasing a variety of habitat that makes this area so rich in birds and animals. Tall ponderosa pines and other conifers support bald eagle nests along this section. An observant paddler will see not only the eagles but their nests as well.

Camping along the shore is not allowed in the wildlife refuge, so paddling on the canoe trail must be a day trip. While some of the lakeshore to the west is publicly owned, camping is difficult because of terrain and vegetation. Most of the shoreline of Klamath Lake is in private ownership, precluding camping. If you paddle far enough up Crystal Creek north of its junction with Recreation Creek, you may be on private land. As long as the channel is navigable and not blocked by structures, you should be okay to paddle.

Camping is sometimes allowed at the launching site at Malone Springs, on USFS land. However, this site is only about 3 miles from Rocky Point, and as such is not positioned well for an overnight destination. If you do decide to camp there, check with the USFS Klamath Ranger District first to make sure regulations have not changed.

Plan to carry all your water in Upper Klamath Lake. While safe to drink if treated, the quality is not good and the taste may be objectionable.

Trip Description

This paddle begins at Rocky Point Resort and Marina, a privately operated resort on a narrow arm of Pelican Bay at the northwest end of Klamath Lake. The resort presently has a restaurant, a small store, RV campsites, and tent campsites. The tent sites are conveniently located at the water's edge. The marina caters mostly to fishermen who seek the giant rainbow trout for which Klamath Lake is famed. It is not primarily a lake that attracts water-skiers. There is also a public launching area a few hundred yards south of the resort, which would be a good alternate place to begin this trip.

From the docks at Rocky Point Marina or the public launch area, turn left and paddle north. Recreation Creek widens into Pelican Bay here, a 0.5-mile-wide bay trending northwest 2 miles from Upper Klamath Lake. The wooded shore on your left is dotted with waterfront vacation homes, each with their own dock. These owners are as interested as you are in privacy and seclusion; generally their in-residence time is quiet and unobtrusive. Within

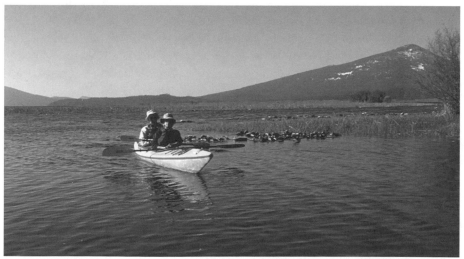

The Crystal Creek canoe trail winds through the National Wildlife Refuge on Klamath Lake's north end

a half mile the number of vacation homes dwindles and you are more able to appreciate the aspen trees and other growth ashore. On your right is the marsh, an impenetrable wall of bullrushes and cattails. Nearly anytime you can hear the characteristic cluck of coots, and in spring the constant trill of red-winged blackbirds. Canada geese paddle away from your boat; marsh wrens flit about. There is no doubt that the marsh is a living place.

Continue north 1 mile from the launch area. You have passed the cabins now, while the channel still parallels the wooded shore but is sometimes separated from it by rushes and small ponds. At the 1-mile point an unmistakable channel opens up leading generally east. This is an 0.8-mile-long shortcut to the Crystal Creek channel, and using this route will shorten paddling distance by 2.5 miles. The canoe trail here (and at other places along the route) is designated by brown signs placed on posts in the water. The information contained on these signs is minimal, usually indicating only that you are on the canoe route. But the signs are helpful in the open-water section of the shortcut.

Continue past the shortcut, following the channel of Recreation Creek. One more mile north (2 miles from launch) you will reach the confluence of Recreation Creek and Crystal Creek. Although you could continue several miles north up Crystal Creek (to where Malone Springs, a boat-launch site accessible from West Side Rd. may allow camping), turn right here and paddle generally south down Crystal Creek. In 1.5 miles, you will reach the open-water area and the east end of the shortcut described earlier. Continue south along the Crystal Creek channel.

Now you are deep in the marsh. Nearly a mile of bullrushes borders you on both sides. It is 2.3 miles south along the Crystal Creek channel to the creek entrance into Pelican Bay. It is impossible to become lost in this area because the channel is so well defined within the marsh. At the entrance to Pelican Bay turn right (north) and, keeping the edge of the marsh on your right, paddle north 1.5 miles to Rocky Point, your launch site.

Alternate or Additional Trips

If you want to increase the length of this trip, consider continuing north in the Crystal Creek channel from its confluence with Recreation Creek. The channel leads north, meandering through the marsh and occasionally approaching the shoreline. Willow stands increase in size and density as you go farther north, providing ideal habitat for beaver. Eventually you will either reach the Crystal Springs area or be stopped by a fence or other barricade on private land. From that turnaround point, backtrack to the Recreation Creek confluence. Before leaving the designated canoe trail, check with administrative agencies for any closures to protect nesting birds.

Besides the Upper Klamath Canoe Trail, the entire expanse of Klamath Lake is available for you to paddle. While you won't find cruising down the middle of this body of water very exciting, shoreline paddling is interesting and fun. One possible trip is to paddle east from Rocky Point, following the north shore of Upper Klamath Lake through the narrows and into adjoining Agency Lake. Agency is less than half the size of Upper Klamath Lake, and much easier to cross. There are two campgrounds: one at Agency Lake Resort, and the other at Williamson River Resort. Private ownership and shoreline characteristics make shoreline camping impractical.

Another trip possibility is to follow the west shore of Upper Klamath Lake south from Rocky Point. For many miles this shore is publicly owned, and camping is allowed if you can find a suitable spot. A steep shoreline and vegetation limit campsites to tiny, make-do places where old logging roads were cut into the banks. Possible sites around an old gravel pit about 5 miles south of Rocky Point are exceptions. Farther south, the shoreline is slightly more hospitable for camping. Be extremely careful with portable stoves along this shore. Campfires are not allowed during the fire season, and are a poor idea at any time in the area.

Other Area Activities

Crater Lake National Park is 30 miles north. Continue north on West Side Rd. to the tiny town of Fort Klamath. Then turn left (north) on Hwy. 62, which leads into the park.

Hiking is popular in two, nearby wilderness areas. Mountain Lakes Wilderness lies a few miles south of Hwy. 140, about 10 miles west of Rocky Point. Trailheads for the Mountain Lakes Wilderness are accessed off Dead Indian Memorial Rd. at Lake of the Woods. You can reach Sky Lakes Wilderness via a gravel road leading to Cold Springs; it turns north from Hwy. 140, 4 miles west of the junction with West Side Rd. It is 11 miles to the trailhead, with the Sky Lakes Wilderness beginning just 0.5 mile from the end of the road.

There are three smaller lakes in the Klamath Lake vicinity that offer interesting day trips in a kayak. Lake of the Woods, Fish Lake, and Fourmile Lake are all reached from Hwy. 140, approximately 10 miles west of Rocky Point.

Contacts

Winema National Forest
Klamath Ranger District
1936 California Ave.
Klamath Falls, OR 97601
(541) 882-7761

U.S. Fish and Wildlife Service
Klamath Basin National Wildlife Refuge
Rt. 1, Box 74
Tulelake, CA 96134
(530) 667-2231

Rocky Point Resort and Marina
(541) 356-2287

Our double kayak floated in the channel, moving almost imperceptibly with the slow current. We were watching a beaver lodge, where wet prints on a peeled log indicated one of the animals had been there recently. We didn't have a lot of hope; a bright, midday sun illuminated everything in crystal-clear relief. Beavers are nocturnal animals, yet something had recently climbed up on that lodge.

A few minutes earlier, a muskrat had swum toward us, its nose above water and beadlike eyes shining as it traced a V-wake directly toward our boat. A few feet away, it decided that we were foreign to the scene and dove beneath us. Five yards beyond us on the other side, the muskrat surfaced and resumed its course, showing us its long bare tail, undulating in the wake. The animal reached shore, turned, and continued parallel to the rushes.

Waiting had stilled the disruption of our paddling. As the creatures around us resumed their routines, we listened to the near-constant cluck of coots in the nearby rushes. Several male blackbirds, vying for dominance in attracting mates, sang loudly from rushes that bent under their weight toward the water. Marsh wrens flitted about tangled clumps of rushes. Counterpoint to the sweetness of birdsong around us was the discordant honk of a raven.

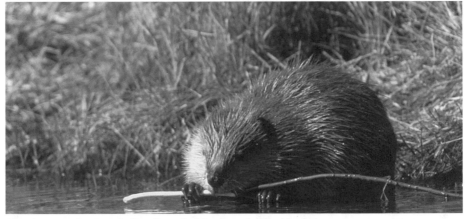

You may spot beavers feeding from their caches of willow bark

Intent upon the beaver lodge, we didn't see the eagle approach. Overhead, we heard the swish of wingbeats so close we could make out the texture of its feathers and the golden eyes that ignored us. Never have we seen a bald eagle so close. No time to point the camera—all we could do was watch as the bird flapped along, then pumped upward toward a 150'-tall pine a hundred yards away on the shore. Her course pinpointed the nest we hadn't noticed and, seconds later, the huge wings folded as she landed on the suspended mass of sticks.

The beaver forgotten, we sat there breathless. As our excitement gradually abated, we turned back to the surroundings. Heading back, we alternately paddled and drifted along. We felt like intruders in the marsh but, at the same time, like a part of it. From now on when we think of Klamath Marsh, the first thing that comes to mind is the sight of that majestic eagle, winging over our boat, just a few paddle lengths away.

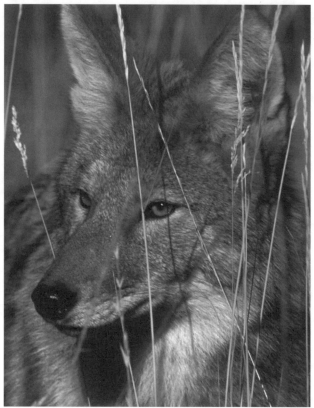

A coyote's serenade is part of the magic of desert camping

PART III.

PACIFIC SOUTHWEST

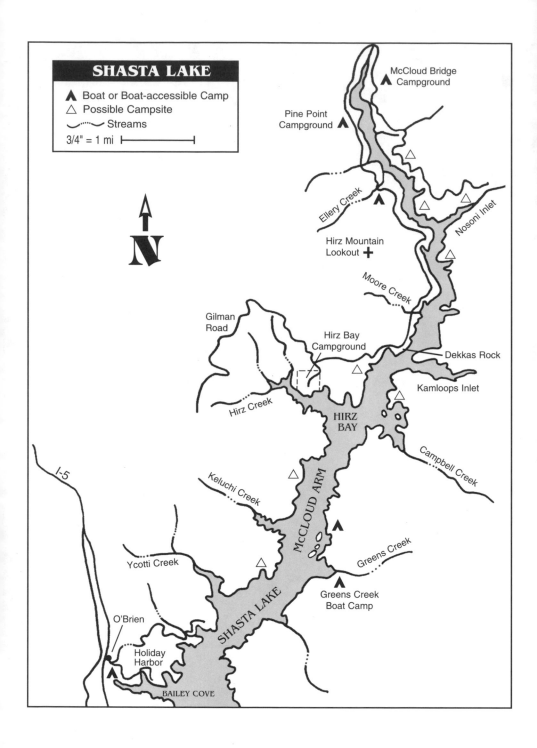

SHASTA LAKE

▲ Boat or Boat-accessible Camp
△ Possible Campsite
⌇⌇ Streams
3/4" = 1 mi ├────────┤

N

McCloud Bridge
Campground

Pine Point
Campground

Ellery Creek

Nosoni Inlet

Hirz Mountain
Lookout ✛

Moore Creek

Gilman
Road

Hirz Bay
Campground

Dekkas Rock

Kamloops Inlet

Hirz Creek

HIRZ
BAY

I-5

Campbell Creek

Keluchi Creek

McCLOUD ARM

Ycotti Creek

Greens Creek

SHASTA LAKE

Greens Creek
Boat Camp

O'Brien

Holiday
Harbor

BAILEY COVE

California

Chapter 9

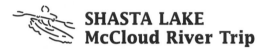

SHASTA LAKE
McCloud River Trip

Trip Details	
Distance:	27 miles
Time:	12 hours paddling
Rating:	Easy
Maps:	USGS 7.5-min: *O'Brien*, *Minnesota Mountain*, and *Bollibokka Mtn*

Summary and Highlights

Shasta Lake is the largest human-made, recreational lake in California. It occupies three major river basins at their confluence: the Sacramento, McCloud, and Pitt. A reservoir built primarily for flood control, it nonetheless provides excellent recreational paddling mainly because it is in a forested area, and the narrow, inundated river valleys offer 370 miles of shoreline. In other words, the lake surface, rather than being a huge body of water, is configured with lots of long, narrow bays and coves. Paddling to explore these inlets is what a kayak trip is all about.

Shoreline camping is allowed on all areas of Shasta Lake, except those posted as closed. This is a major factor in making adventure kayaking, and especially overnight camping, possible here. A permit from the U.S. Forest Service is required when using USFS launching or parking facilities.

The trip described here begins at a very accessible resort and campground area, and passes up the narrow McCloud Arm of the lake, to the inflow. It can be done in two days, with one overnight camp, or very easily for nonhardened paddlers in three days, camping out for two nights. The route passes by small islands, limestone outcroppings, dense forest, and many bays and coves. The area is popular with recreational users who spend time on house-boats, water skis, and personal watercraft.

When to go: You can paddle on Shasta Lake any time of the year, but doing so is most enjoyable from early spring to late fall. The lake does not freeze over in the winter. Water levels are lowest in late winter, when the reservoir is drawn down for hydroelectric generation, or lowered to provide storage room for flood control. Spring runoff brings the lake up to full-pool level if sufficient precipitation has occurred. Water levels then remain relatively constant through early summer, dropping considerably by fall. Temperatures are mild beginning in mid-April, grow quite warm during the summer, and moderate again in mid-September.

For the paddler, one factor in scheduling a trip on Shasta Lake is minimizing conflict with other recreational users. A number of marinas on the lake rent houseboats, with many hundreds in the total fleet. Good launching

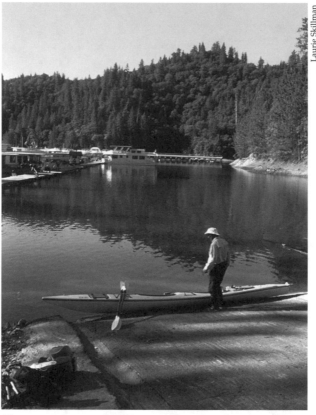

There are numerous launch ramps at various locations, like this one at Holiday Harbor Resort

ramps, giving access even when the lake is 50 feet or more below full, mean that waterskiers and other powerboat users find the lake, with its comparatively warm waters, appealing. Rarely will you be the only boat on the water on Shasta Lake.

To avoid the worst crowds, don't go on weekends, and especially avoid holidays. A paddle during the week will avoid most congestion. Houseboat rentals are usually for a weekend, or for a full week. You will share with the latter renters, but not the former. A great time on Shasta Lake is early in the season, before June 15. The lake will be high, and summer vacationers won't yet be on the water.

Hazards: Shasta Lake water is not unusually cold, except early season near the inflow of each arm when the rivers bring in snowmelt. By early summer, the water temperature has increased, and hypothermia is not as great a danger as in some other lakes. However, remember that prolonged immersion can be dangerous, even in water above 60°.

Because of the heavy use, Shasta Lake water must be considered unsafe for drinking. The same goes for any tributary streams, or springs, which you may find. Filter, treat, or boil all water here. Many established campgrounds have water systems developed by the Forest Service, and such sources provide safe, potable water.

Wind must also be considered a hazard on Shasta, as on any body of water. However, the shoreline is so irregular that there are always sheltered spots nearby. Waiting out a sudden onslaught of wind waves at an unintended destination in a small cove or bay should be considered part of kayaking.

Bears are very numerous around Shasta Lake. Many are skilled at obtaining food from campers, so be sure to bear-bag your food, hanging it well out of reach. Don't put it in your kayak. Any respectable bear can tear open a kayak as easily as we open a paper bag.

Rattlesnakes are present in the area. Keep a watch when you go ashore, and look your intended campsite over carefully. Watch also for poison oak, which is widespread.

How to Get There

Shasta Lake is in Northern California, 14 miles north of Redding accessed by I-5. Turn at the O'Brien exit, north 3 miles from the bridge that crosses the lake, and follow the signs to Bailey Cove Camp.

Area Features, Background, and Tips

Shasta Lake, keystone of the huge Central Valley Project in California, was created when Shasta Dam was built between 1935 and 1945. This dam is the second largest and tallest concrete dam in the country. The reservoir behind it ranks as the largest human-made impoundment in California.

Little modern history was destroyed by the 30,000-acre inundation when the dam was filled. A major pioneer trail to Oregon passed along the Sacramento River, and was followed later by the railroad. The portion of this route beneath the lake was lost, as were several copper mining locations. Today, the only remains of the copper mines in the area are on the Squaw Creek Arm.

Perhaps the most significant loss was the archaeology sites. Native Americans used the Shasta area heavily. The rivers offered abundant salmon runs, while the surrounding country was rich in game. The hills provided various berries, acorns, and pine nuts. Permanent village sites, as well as fishing and foraging camps, were flooded by the rising waters of Shasta Lake.

Shasta is a low-elevation lake, reaching up narrow, forested river valleys, and providing very mild conditions in an area that has the appearance of being at much greater altitude. True, the forest is mixed-species, with lots of oaks, some maples, and cottonwoods interspersed with digger pines, knobcone pines, ponderosa pines, and firs. The modest 1,067' elevation also allows temperatures to rise during high-pressure systems in the summer; days are often warmer than 100°F, and sometimes as high as 115°.

Limestone is the rock most often exposed, especially along the McCloud Arm of the lake. It was formed when the area was beneath the sea. Deposition of undersea creatures formed the beds, which were later buried deeply, subjected to great heat and pressure, and metamorphosed into limestone. Later, the undersea beds were uplifted to where we see them today as weathered, sharp-edged cliffs or peaks. The dissolving action of water on the limestone erodes it in uneven patterns; small ridges are left projecting above as the rest of the surface dissolves. These ridges can become knife-sharp. Shasta Caverns, a large cave attraction on the east shore of the McCloud Arm, is a classic limestone cave formed as water, flowing through cracks and fissures, slowly dissolved the limestone.

The different arms of Shasta Lake display varying features, aura, and character. Fortunately, the use of motorized craft is heaviest in the western arms of the lake. Fishing is perhaps the major attraction in the eastern arms. This means that paddling will be more enjoyable on the McCloud River, Squaw Creek, and Pitt River arms, all on the east side of the lake.

All inland waters are areas of environmental concern, whether declared by an agency or not. This is just as true on Shasta, where the great size of the lake may tempt some to be less careful about sanitation than on a smaller lake. Pack out all your litter, including your human waste if you can't always use the toilets provided.

There are 11 private marinas on Shasta Lake. In addition, the Forest Service maintains 6 launching facilities with parking areas, 17 developed campgrounds, 4 shoreline camps, and 4 boat-access camps on the lake. But the rugged country, ragged shoreline, and great size of the lake, broken as it is into five separate arms, seems to distance these facilities from one another.

Trip Description

Launch at Bailey Cove Camp, a Forest Service campground with seven sites, in the O'Brien area 17 miles north of Redding on Interstate 5. As an alternative, Holiday Harbor Resort has an RV Park and campground nearby, as well as launching facilities at the resort. All of these facilities are located in Bailey Cove, a mile-long inlet on the west side of the McCloud Arm. The ferry taking tourists to Shasta Caverns also leaves from Bailey Cove. Paddle east out of the cove into the main arm. You can see the road to the caverns high up on the east shore of the arm, and also the ferry's docking facility.

Turn left (north) and in 1 mile, you reach the Lakeview Marina Resort on the west shore. The marina is easily identified by the docking facilities. Continue 0.5 mile past the marina and you will be opposite the mile-long narrow cove at the entrance to Ycotti Creek. North 0.6 mile from this cove, on the southwest side of a rounded projecting point, is a passable campsite (2.5 miles from launch). One mile directly east, in a wide cove on the east shore, is Greens Creek Boat Camp, a Forest Service boat-access campground with eight sites and toilets. Camping is free year-round at this beautiful, peaceful site.

North of Greens Creek 0.5 mile, three islands (at full pool) provide interest and a possible stopover site. Opposite the islands, on the west shore, is a 0.6-mile-long cove at Keluche Creek. One mile north of the islands, on the west shore just past an unnamed creek, are a couple of possible campsites. Continue north from the unnamed creek 1 mile to Hirz Bay. Hirz Bay, a 1.3-mile-long inlet on the west shore is accessed by car from Gilman Road, and has launching facilities and a Forest Service campground.

Opposite Hirz Bay, on the east shore, is a delightful 0.7-mile-deep bay formed by the Campbell Creek confluence. Several private cabins are located along shore in the south portion of the bay. Two small islands add to its ambiance. Possible campsites may be found just north of the peninsula forming the north pincer of the bay (6 miles from launch).

Back on the west shore, 0.3 mile north of Hirz Bay, are possible campsites on a tiny point which juts several hundred feet out in an easterly, then a southerly, direction. Continue north 0.7 mile along the west shore to Dekkas Rock. Camping possibilities look good here, but you would have to share the area with campers who have come in along Gilman Road. This is a group camp. Opposite Dekkas Rock, on the east shore, is enchanting 1-mile-long Kamloops Inlet. There are good camping possibilities on various rounded points within the inlet; houseboats prefer to tie up in the heads of coves between points. Paddle 1 mile up-lake from Dekkas Rock to Mathles Creek, entering from the east. There is a possible campsite on the north point of the tiny Mathles cove (8.5 miles from launch).

Up-lake 0.3 mile from Mathles Creek, on the west shore, is Moore Creek, a developed Forest Service campground. If you carry your water, replenish your containers here. Continuing 0.6 mile up-lake, there is a possible campsite at an indent in the broad point just north of Dooles Creek on the east shore. One-half mile north of Dooles Creek is a delightful, narrow inlet where Nosoni Creek enters, also on the east shore. There is a possible campsite at the

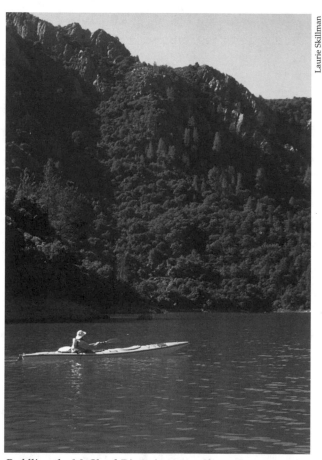

Laurie Skillman

Paddling the McCloud River Arm near Shasta Caverns and Bailey Cove

end of the north entrance point of the inlet (10 miles from launch). This inlet has a trail along its north shore from Ferry Road, 1 mile east. For several miles up-lake and down-lake from this spot, the views have been dominated by Hirz Mountain on the west side of the arm. The Forest Service lookout on the summit is over 3,000 feet in elevation, about 2,000 feet above the water level.

Paddle north 0.7 mile from Nosoni Creek to a very narrow 0.3-mile-long inlet on the east shore. This inlet abuts Ferry Road. Continue north 0.5 mile from the narrow inlet to Ellery Creek, a Forest Service camp on the west shore. North of Ellery Creek 1 mile along the west shore is another Forest Service camp at Pine Point. The McCloud Arm makes a decided bend around Pine Point, and once you have paddled past this bend, you can see McCloud Bridge, just 1 mile up-lake. There is a Forest Service camp of the same name at McCloud Bridge (13.5 miles from launch), but this is a fee camp and usually very popular. Look on the east shore, several hundred yards south of the campground, for a gently sloping shoreline where you can camp.

As you paddle north up the ever-narrowing arm from McCloud Bridge, you will reach an area where the lake ends and river current begins. Exactly where this transformation occurs depends upon the level of Shasta Lake. If lower water levels prevent you from reaching McCloud Bridge, this paddle will end for you at one of the camps you passed as you paddled north along the McCloud Arm. To return to your launch site, retrace the route you paddled.

Alternate or Additional Trips

Obviously, on a body of water as extensive as Shasta Lake, there are many possible trips. It is neither my intent to detail these trips here nor have I paddled them all. But you can easily design your own trip with nothing more than a chart of the lake. Shorter or much longer trips than the one described are easy to route. Keep in mind that the eastern arms offer more forested shores, and powerboat traffic is somewhat less in the eastern regions.

Much of the Pitt River Arm was not cleared of forest prior to inundation, and as a result there are lots of snags and dead trees in the water. This has enhanced fishing. Waterskiing is not allowed up-lake from Browns Canyon on the Pitt Arm, providing miles of narrow fjordlike lake that is free of ski activity. However, possible campsites in the narrow section are quite limited. Down-lake from Browns Canyon, the shore topography is less steep, and the flatter terrain offers many good camping possibilities.

The Squaw Creek Arm has lots of wide, shallow inlets, a result of gentler terrain. Campsites are easy to find in the Squaw Creek Arm. In some areas, at full pool, nearly every knoll and point offers a pleasant campsite. As the water level drops, it becomes more difficult to camp under trees, which might be some distance from the water.

Other Area Activities

While there are hiking trails in many places around Shasta Lake, consider the hot, dry nature of the region before taking serious hikes. Taking plenty of water is the key to hiking safely here. Try the trails at Bailey Cove, Packers Bay, Hirz Bay, Jones Valley, or Shasta Dam.

A visit to Shasta Caverns is worth experiencing. This limestone cavern is reached by crossing the McCloud Arm by ferry, then taking a bus up to the cavern entrance, high on a limestone hillside. A fee is charged. Remember that this cavern is not the only cave system in the Shasta area, it is just one of several that has been *found*. There are undoubtedly others that haven't been discovered yet, or else lie flooded beneath the water.

Samwell Cave is located on the east shore of the McCloud Arm, a short distance south of McCloud Bridge. It opens out from a limestone promontory that overlooks the lake. The cave is protected by a locked gate. The key, and a necessary permit, can be obtained at Shasta Lake Visitor Information Center.

Contacts

For comprehensive information about the Shasta-Trinity area, maps, and permits, contact:

Shasta-Trinity National Forests
Supervisor's Office
2400 Washington Ave.
Redding, CA 96001
(530) 246-5222

Specific information on water levels and conditions at Shasta Lake, as well as status of campgrounds, facilities, and permits, can be obtained from:

Shasta Lake Ranger District
14225 Holiday Drive
Redding, CA 96003
(530) 275-1589

Shasta Lake Visitor Information Center
(530) 275-1589

Holiday Harbor Resort, in Bailey Cove, is mentioned as an alternate launch spot for the trip described in this chapter. The phone at Holiday Harbor Resort is (530) 238-2383.

We paddled out past the rafts of houseboats moored in Bailey Cove, our double kayak the only muscle-powered craft in sight. We left the 5-knot, no-wake area around the marina (our passage had caused no disturbance), and headed north into the McCloud Arm, glassy smooth in the early morning stillness. An osprey passed close by, pumping along on irregular wingbeats. On the east shore, several vultures sat on a driftwood log, wings outspread to catch the early sun.

An hour later and some 3 miles north, we were passed by the first powerboat of the morning, moving up-lake near the opposite shore. The presence of another boat was not disconcerting. We continued paddling north, exploring first the east, and then the west shores as we went.

Live oaks, an occasional madrone, and thin digger pines with bluish-green needles carpet the shore. Occasional small stands of knobcone pines raise trunks clustered tightly with cones. The forest is not open; brush is the rule where competing trees have not shaded it out. A deer in its red, summer coat looks up before slipping surreptitiously into a thicket. At full pool now, there is little to reveal that Shasta Lake is a reservoir and not a natural lake with a stationary water level. In one cove is a belted kingfisher, claiming domain from a dry limb near the water. In the next, a great blue heron rules from his wading position in the bight; unsure as we come into view, he comments with a loud squawk before slowly flapping away.

Later, in Kamloops Inlet, where a speed limit takes the fun out of things for power-boaters, we paddle peacefully along. A few houseboats have taken up temporary residence in coves, but their occupants are not those who are here to tear around in jet skis. It was easy to find a tiny secluded cove, where a dip in the lake water (just the right temperature) was very refreshing. Later, a tree-studded knoll, sloping back gently from shore, beckons as a lunch stop. We land, then find a shady spot to sit and eat, and contemplate where we are. Our kayak makes it easy to find solitude, whether coming upon an unoccupied camping area, or poking into nooks and crannies where we are alone.

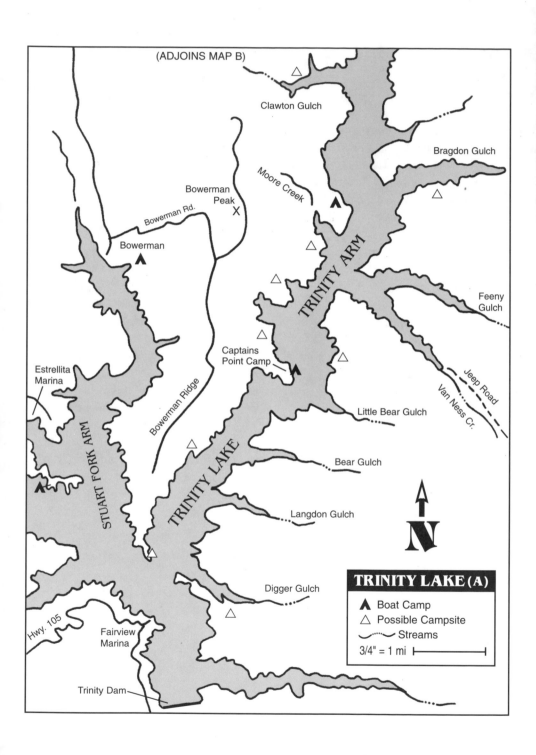

(ADJOINS MAP B)

Clawton Gulch

Bragdon Gulch

Moore Creek

Bowerman
Peak
X

Bowerman Rd.

Bowerman

TRINITY ARM

Feeny
Gulch

Estrellita
Marina

Bowerman Ridge

Captains
Point Camp

Little Bear Gulch

Van Ness Cr.

Jeep Road

STUART FORK ARM

TRINITY LAKE

Bear Gulch

Langdon Gulch

N

Digger Gulch

TRINITY LAKE (A)

🅰 Boat Camp
△ Possible Campsite
⌒⌒ Streams
3/4" = 1 mi ├────────┤

Hwy. 105

Fairview
Marina

Trinity Dam

California

Chapter 10

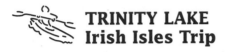 **TRINITY LAKE**
Irish Isles Trip

Trip Details

Distance:	25 miles
Time:	12 hours paddling
Rating:	Moderate
Maps:	USGS 7.5-min: *Trinity Dam*, *Trinity Center*, and *Papoose Creek*

Summary and Highlights

This two-day paddle on beautiful Trinity Lake (also known as Clair Engle Lake) is rated "Moderate" for two reasons: the distance traveled, and the possibility of adverse paddling conditions because of wind and wind waves. Extend the trip to three days on the water and the rating changes to "Easy," because more time is available to wait out any adverse conditions, and there is less distance to be paddled each day.

Trinity Lake is striking, nestled as it is in narrow canyons with densely forested shorelines. From many places on the water the majestic snowcaps of the Trinity Alps can be seen, rising above the closer mountains surrounding the lake. While the lake is actually a reservoir, it resembles the coastal fjords of southeast Alaska, an impression that only slightly diminishes when water levels drop below the high watermark.

The steep, wooded topography surrounding the lake makes finding a spot to land a kayak challenging. The same is true of finding a place to camp. There is one boat-in Forest Service camp along the route of this trip, but its location (close to the launch point) makes it awkward to use. We have care-

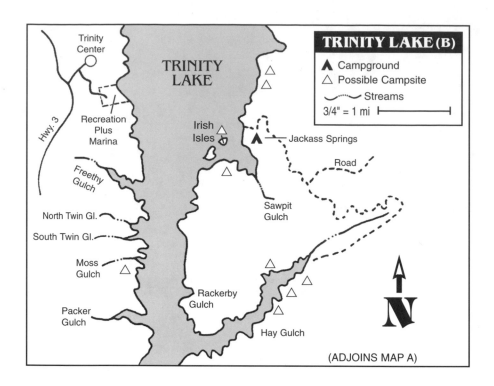

fully scouted other possible campsites, and note their location in the trip description.

Irish Isles, the destination of this trip, are two islands, one of which is heavily wooded, steep, and becomes a peninsula when the water level drops a few feet. The other is an idyllic islet about a hundred yards across, offering three unimproved campsites. The isle's beaches are clean gravel and inviting, its conifers provide shade, and its orientation offers views out across a broad bay backed by the Trinity Alps. If the three sites are occupied, there are alternative sites on the mainland nearby.

At 2,370' elevation when full, Trinity Lake is high enough to avoid excessive summer heat, yet low enough that the lake does not freeze in winter. This medium elevation makes possible the lush forest environment along the shoreline.

While there is considerable recreational use of powerboats and houseboats on Trinity Lake, the size of the impoundment, its elevation, and its somewhat out-of-the-way location keep these pressures from being extreme. Most of the powered recreation takes place on the western arms of the lake. The main arm along the Trinity River Valley is less traveled. It also boasts many long, narrow inlets for the kayaker to explore.

When to go: Late spring and early summer, before lake levels drop, offer rewarding experiences to the kayaker. Check with the USFS to ascertain the lake level. If you paddle when the water is low, the established campground and the possible campsites described in this book may be several feet above the water. One positive result is that low-water conditions will uncover new camping areas. If you prefer camps with shade trees, just portage up your gear.

Hazards: Water in Trinity Lake is cold in the early season when the lake is filling with snowmelt. The water warms up quite a bit later in the summer but the usual caveats about cold water, and the undesirability of unintended immersion in it, are appropriate here.

Plan to paddle early in the day to avoid winds, which may develop in the afternoon.

This is black bear country, and there is the possibility of encountering a habituated bear around established camps. Be sure to bear-bag your food, whether you are in an established camp or on your own at a seldom-visited point.

Rattlesnakes are not numerous around Trinity Lake. Still, be cautious and look around before stepping ashore or setting up camp.

How to Get There

From I-5 in Redding, California, turn west toward the coast on Hwy. 299. Drive approximately 30 miles on 299 to the junction with Hwy. 105, which leads right (north) to Lewiston, Lewiston Dam, Trinity Dam, and Trinity Lake. Turn right on 105 and proceed 4 miles north to Lewiston, then continue north 5 miles along Lewiston Lake to Trinity Lake. You reach the Fairview launching area 1 mile north of Trinity Dam off the main (and only) paved road.

Area Features, Background, and Tips

The Trinity Lake area lies just east of the Trinity Alps, a mountain range that is actually a part of the Klamath Mountains, lying inland from the coast in northern California and southern Oregon. Because rainfall is abundant and winters are mild, many plant species that in less hospitable areas are separated by temperature and latitude grow side by side here. A short distance from the lake cradled in the "Alps" are active glaciers, a rarity this close to a coast at this latitude. The area around the lake exudes wilderness, and indeed the Trinity Lake segment of the Whiskeytown-Shasta-Trinity National Recreation Area abuts the vast Trinity Alps Wilderness.

The area is unusual in terms of its geology. About 350 million years ago the area was under the sea, receiving sediments from the western edge of the

North American continent. Sea life perished and settled to the ocean floor. As the milleniums passed, this sediment built up and its pressure changed clays to shale, sand into sandstone, and marine skeletons into limestone. Uplift followed by inundation was a repeating cycle.

Plate movement about 150 million years ago brought a period of mountain building. Heat and pressure metamorphozed shale into slate, and converted other sedimentary and volcanic rocks to quartzite, gneiss, and schist. In colliding with the North American plate, the Pacific plate was forced deep beneath the continent. Massive piles of scrapings from ancient sea floors and adjoining formations resulted in the great variety of rocks and soils we see here today. The subducted Pacific plate melted, sending magma rising upward—much of it cooling before reaching the surface and forming granite.

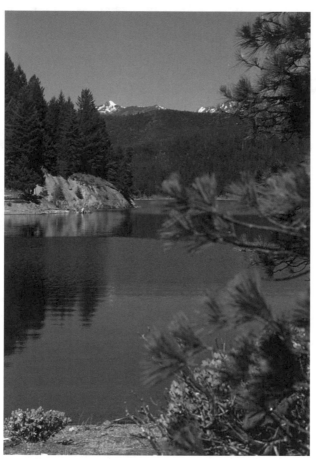

Irish Isles offer pines for shade beside gravel beaches, and a magnificent view of the snowcapped Trinity Alps

Around 50 million years ago the Klamath range was uplifted above the reach of the sea. Glacial action and water erosion have shaped the landscape we see today in the Trinity Valley.

Factor in the mild climate, moderate elevation, and Coast Range location, and it is no wonder that this region is a recreation paradise. Wildflowers here can be spectacular. You may see checkermallow, fireweed, tiger lily, white clover, owl clover, Indian paintbrush, cascade lily, narrow goldenrod, lupine, azure penstemon, shooting star, crimson columbine, larkspur, Mariposa lily, skyrocket, cow parsnip, wandering daisy, and many others, depending upon the season. At any one time, some have finished blooming and others have not yet begun.

The forests are mostly mixed conifers, including ponderosa pine (with Jeffrey pine at higher elevations), sugar pine, western white pine, incense cedar, Shasta fir, white fir, and Douglas-fir, varying with elevation and aspect. Damp areas nourish big leaf maple and cottonwoods. Willows and alders cluster in riparian areas. Oaks are present in favorable locations at the lower elevations.

As you might expect, such a vast area of prime habitat nurtures a variety of wildlife. Birds are plentiful, and from your kayak you can expect to see great blue herons, kingfishers, green-back herons, an occasional black-crowned night heron, as well as ospreys and bald eagles. Ravens are also quite common. You may also see any of several woodpeckers that live in forest habitats. Jays, juncos, robins and other thrushes, as well as sparrows, warblers, and other families are common, depending upon the season and their migratory patterns.

The largest animal is the elk, not plentiful but occasionally present. Next in size is the black bear, which is abundant. There are deer in nearly every location. Mountain lions are present but almost never seen. Coyotes, bobcats, and small forest animals all prey heavily on many different rodents. When camping within this complex ecosystem, remember to bear-bag your food if you don't want to upset the food web.

Trinity Dam and Lewiston Dam—both on the Trinity River—were completed in 1961 and are part of the huge Central Valley Project, which was designed to deliver both electricity and water to central and southern California. Water is diverted at Lewiston Dam through an 11-mile-long tunnel into Whiskeytown Lake, just a few miles west of Redding. Here, hydroelectric generation is again possible as water is released into a huge canal system on its way to the Sacramento-San Joaquin delta and metropolitan areas. Sacrificing a fine anadromous fishery in the upper Trinity River, and inundating a unique valley rich in local history, for power generation and water supply has been a controversial trade-off.

The Forest Service has developed four boat-in campgrounds on Trinity Lake; these have toilets but no water. In addition there are half a dozen campgrounds that are on the lakeshore and accessed by road. There are other campgrounds away from the lake under the auspices of the recreation area, besides several private facilities. Camping along the lakeshore is allowed, as long as the particular area has not been closed. Checking with rangers is the best bet here, for closures vary by season and location. Casual supplies may be purchased either at the resorts or in Trinity Center, the community on Highway 3 near the north end of Trinity Lake, on the west shore. If you launch in any of the Forest Service facilities, you will need both launch and parking permits, which are available at the resort.

Trip Description

Put in at the Fairview launch ramp, which shares an access road with Trinity Alps Marina, off the main road north 1 mile from Trinity Dam. Launch and parking permits may be purchased at the marina. The point which you see due north of you is the south end of Bowerman Ridge, which forms a mountainous, peninsular boundary between the Stuart Fork Arm of the lake to the west, and the Trinity Arm running north-northeast. Take a wind check, then paddle north 0.7 mile across to the point of Bowerman Ridge. Note that camping is possible at several spots on the narrow point.

Directly east from Bowerman Point is the entrance to Digger Gulch, an inlet trending southeast for 1 mile from the east shore. A 5-mile-per-hour speed zone is in effect for the area around the head of Digger Gulch. From the entrance to Digger Gulch, paddle north 1 mile up the Trinity Arm to the entrance to Langdon Gulch, also a mile-long inlet in the east shore. Continue north 0.8 mile in the arm to a third inlet along the east shore; this one is Bear Gulch (2.7 miles from launch). Northwest of Bear Gulch inlet, across the arm on the west shore, is a small cove just a hundred yards or so long. The head of this cove is split by two, small rounded points. Camping possibilities are present here for those who search.

Leaving Bear Gulch, paddle 1 mile up-lake, passing a sharp point around which the arm bends 90° in an easterly direction. The sizable inlet at the outside of this bend, due north of the point, contains no feasible campsites, at least at full-pool level. Paddle east 1 mile beyond the sharp point, to the entrance of Little Bear Gulch. Here, the main arm turns north again. Note that Captains Point boat-in camp is incorrectly shown on some maps as being at the south end of the rounded peninsula on the west shore, across from Little Bear Gulch (this is the peninsula causing the arm to do all the bending in this spot). Actually, Captains Point boat camp is located on the northwest point of this peninsula (4.5 miles from launch).

Continuing north past Captains Point boat camp, notice that the east shore to the east-northeast is broken into a series of small coves divided by points. There are camping possibilities on two of these points. On the west shore, 0.6 mile north of Captains Point boat camp, is the entrance to a forked inlet which is 0.5 mile long. Good camping possibilities exist on the south entrance point, part way into the inlet. Paddle north 0.5 mile from the unnamed, forked inlet to another 0.3-mile-long inlet on the west shore. It may be possible to camp at the back of this cove.

Paddle northeast 0.5 mile to the entrance of a long inlet on the east shore. This inlet is forked; the north branch is Feeny Creek and the south branch is Van Ness Creek, where a jeep road descends to the water. Both Feeny and Van Ness creek gulches are 5-mile-per-hour speed zones from their confluence to the stream inlets. Stroke your way north 1 mile, passing Moore Creek inlet on the west shore on the way, to the entrance of Bragdon Gulch, a 1.5-mile-long inlet on the east shore (7 miles from launch). Bragdon Gulch is a pleasant spot; there is a possible campsite on a prominent, rounded point on the south shore, 1 mile from the inlet mouth.

Go north 1 mile from Bragdon Gulch, to the mouth of an unnamed inlet on the east shore. This 0.5-mile-long inlet trends eastward before turning 90° North. Continue 0.8 mile past the unnamed inlet to the mouth of Clawton Gulch on the west shore. Clawton offers some interesting side coves at full-pool level. One mile north of Clawton, Hay Gulch leads northeast 2 miles from the east shore of the arm (8.8 miles from launch). There are several camping possibilities on points in the last 0.5 mile of this gulch.

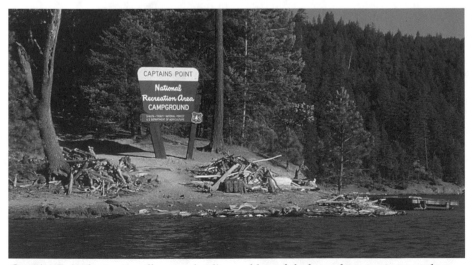

Captains Point boat camp offers easy landing and lots of shade—welcome on summer days

From the mouth of Hay Gulch, paddle north 0.8 mile up the arm to Rackerby Gulch on the east shore, passing Packer Gulch on the west shore in the process. One-half mile north of Rackerby, Moss Gulch lies on the west shore. Not a long inlet that you would particularly notice, it is formed by a "hammerhead"-shaped point at the north entrance, where there are great camping sites. North of Moss Gulch within 0.5 mile, you pass North Twin and South Twin gulches on the west shore. One-half mile farther north, Freethy Gulch forms a 0.5-mile-long inlet in the west shore (11.5 miles from launch).

Across from Freethy Gulch along the east shore, paddle north 1 mile to the Irish Isles. The southernmost, which you reach first, is the largest at some 300 yards across, and is heavily timbered with steep shorelines on its west and south sides. The north isle, separated from the south isle by 200-300 feet of water at full pool, is one third its sister's size with a lighter smattering of trees. There are three camping possibilities, one on each point of the triangular-shaped islet. The fine-gravel beaches are gently sloping at full pool, offering good swimming and easy landing. The western views from these campsites are fantastic. The Trinity Arm of the lake broadens here to 1.5 miles and more; the backdrop is the snowcapped Trinity Alps.

If the Irish Isles sites are being used, possible campsites can be found on points on either shore of Sawpit Gulch, southeast 0.5 mile from Irish Isles.

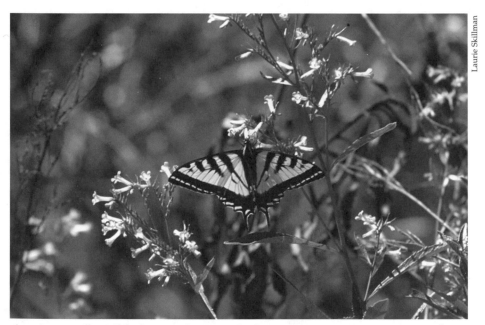

Laurie Skillman

A western swallowtail feeds on a todos santos bush

Jackass Springs, a Forest Service camp accessible by road, is 0.7 mile north of the isles on the east shore. North 0.25 mile farther along the east shore are camping possibilities on two gently-sloping points. To return to the Fairview launch facility, retrace the route you just paddled.

Alternate Trips

Many variations on the described trip can be made on Trinity Lake. For a leisurely day trip or an overnight that involves only 4 miles of paddling, launch at Recreation Plus Marina southeast of Trinity Center and paddle approximately 2 miles southeast to the Irish Isles. By utilizing Captains Point boat camp, or any of the suggested campsites described in this chapter, you can design trips of longer duration, camping in various spots. The combinations depend upon available time and your skills at finding campsites.

Additional Trips

Lewiston Lake, immediately downriver from Trinity Dam, is a narrow, attractive 5-mile-long body of water, which is quite interesting. A speed limit is in effect here, minimizing disturbance from anglers who use motors. The lake is a catchment for water released from the Trinity power plant, and also diverts water to the Central Valley Project. Even though formed by a dam and technically a reservoir, the water level in Lewiston is nearly constant. Yet, flow levels vary with releases from the power plant, and the narrow configuration of the lake means that there is a varying current, depending upon the width and depth of the lake at any given point. Steady water levels have helped trees and riparian plants colonize the shore, as well as several islands within the lake. Lewiston is a beautiful lake with 15 miles of wooded shoreline, providing prime habitat for waterbirds, including many songbirds. Several marsh areas add to the attractiveness for wildlife. Along Hwy. 105, which parallels the lake on the west, are three Forest Service campgrounds with access to Lewiston Lake, in addition to a private RV park.

Should you decide to paddle Lewiston, it will be an experience you're not likely to forget. Be sure to do your paddling in a downstream direction, because the current makes it difficult to paddle upstream. Also remember that the water is very cold, due to its release from the bottom of Trinity Lake.

Whiskeytown Lake, on Hwy. 299 just a few miles west of Redding, is also part of the Central Valley Project, and administered by the Park Service. Paddling this lake makes a very enjoyable day trip. Pine groves and rounded boulders dot the shore, adding beauty to the paddling experience. The ambience is much like a lake in the Sierra.

Other Area Activities

Visit Trinity Center, relocated from its historic location that is now beneath the lake. While there, take in the private collection at the Scott Museum, which contains memorabilia from the early days in the Trinity area. Weaverville, the historic seat of Trinity County, lies a short distance southwest where Hwy. 3 joins Hwy. 299. The Jake Jackson Museum downtown portrays the early days in the area. The Joss House, also in Weaverville, is the oldest continuously used Chinese Taoist Temple in California, now administered as a California state park.

Another major attraction for outdoors enthusiasts is the trail system in the Trinity Alps Wilderness just west of Trinity Lake. Several different trailheads take hikers and backpackers to routes leading to peaks, glaciers, mountain lakes, and meadows. The heavy snowfall in the area often postpones the hiking season to late June at the higher elevations.

Contacts

Shasta-Trinity National Forests
2400 Washington Ave.
Redding, CA 96001
(530) 246-5222

Weaverville Ranger District
PO Box 1190
Weaverville, CA 96093
(530) 623-2121

The disturbance ahead was drawing our attention as we paddled up the narrow, Trinity Lake Arm. The raucous calls of complaining ravens grew louder as we approached. Then we saw an osprey pair, one hovering near their nest at the top of a tall snag, while the other swooped, dove, and flapped after the ravens. There would be no pillaging by the black scavengers as long as the osprey were near the nest.

Later a great blue heron pumped by, progressing not much faster then we were against the afternoon breeze. A red-breasted sapsucker curved down and then up, landing on the trunk of small oak on the shore. Nearby, clusters of migrating swallow-tailed butterflies swarmed around a clump of flowering deer bush. In the next cove, a black-crowned night heron, who glared at us with baleful orange eyes, decided to stay on its perch in an alder. Beneath the tree a previously unseen family of American mergansers squawked in unison, then took to the air, circled, and landed behind us.

Perhaps it was the sheltered location that caused the wildlife concentration, because nearly an hour passed before we saw another creature. But the beautiful lake was reward enough. The breeze was steady in our faces but varying at the inlets, so that the water surface was a patchwork of riffles and small waves—confused, non-threatening. We paddled on, watching the trees move by. With two hours to reach our camp, there was no need to hurry.

We knew that Trinity Lake is more noted for its scenery than wildlife. But we had seen more than our share of creatures. The sun dropped lower as we approached the cove where we were to camp. Then we were in the shadow of the steep mountain that forms the shore. Sheltered here, the water was smooth and reflective as we paddled the last mile. We became reflective, too, replaying in our minds what we had seen out on the lake that morning. An osprey stooped to the surface, caught a fish, and headed for shore. All went well until a bald eagle, dropping from above like a missile, began harrying the osprey. The osprey swerved, turned, and swooped with the eagle in pursuit. With the persistent eagle gaining, the osprey finally dropped its meal; the eagle caught the fish in midair. It hardly seemed fair.

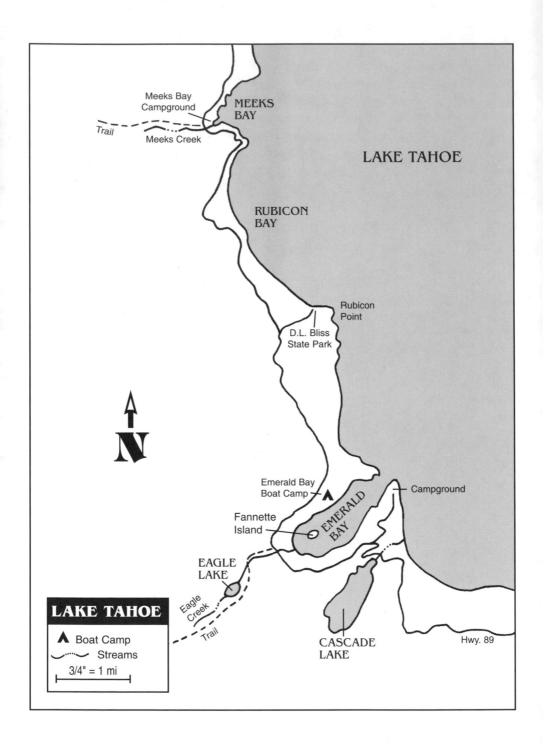

California

Chapter 11

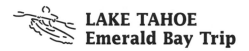

LAKE TAHOE
Emerald Bay Trip

Trip Details	
Distance:	12 miles
Time:	5 hours paddling
Rating:	Easy to Moderate
Maps:	USGS 7.5-min: *Meeks Bay* and *Emerald Bay*

Summary and Highlights

Tahoe needs no introduction as a destination for land-based pursuits, but as a sea-kayaking waterway it's another matter. Nowhere in the western U.S. can you paddle in waters seeming more pristine than at Lake Tahoe (unless you portage your boat down into Crater Lake and secure permission to paddle). At Tahoe you can still see the granite-sand bottom under your kayak at 50' depths, and watch the water turn cobalt when you reach really deep water. Deep water is nearby; on this trip there are places within yards of shore where you have more than 1,000 feet of water under your boat. This trip begins at the National Forest campground at Meeks Bay on the west shore, and features paddling a two-day round trip with an overnight at the Emerald Bay Boat Camp, the only exclusive boat camp on the lake. Without question this route showcases the most spectacular scenery at Lake Tahoe.

Tahoe is big, and the area is heavily populated. By paddling your kayak early in the morning, you can witness the sunrise from water level, or keep abreast of a family of mergansers at the water's edge, and be surprisingly alone. Powerboats don't skim along close to the shore, where huge, underwater boulders, sandy bottoms, and wildlife make your paddle an endless variety of experiences. Midday near a popular marina—especially over the weekend during high season—you cannot avoid close company with power-boats. This trip was carefully chosen to avoid many of those high-usage spots, and allow you to experience a little bit of the Tahoe that was. The route also passes by state park land for one third the distance, showcases vertical gran-ite cliffs plunging underwater to great depths, and allows you to take in the grandeur of glacier-carved Emerald Bay from water level. Complete solitude will elude you on this trip but other benefits will make up for it. After your trip, Tahoe will never seem the same to you; it will mean much more.

When to go: Tahoe doesn't freeze in normal winters; there is too much vol-ume and current for that. But late-fall snows close most of the lakeside busi-nesses and make access to many places next to impossible. Access to Meeks Bay Campground is usually possible by mid-May, but the facilities won't open for another month. Lingering snows may make the opening of the Emerald Bay Boat Camp an early June event. From a practical standpoint, the paddling season runs from June through September. Nights at Tahoe are nearly always chilly, especially in spring and fall. Days during the summer can be warm, but not too hot because of the elevation of 6,200 feet.

Hazards: You must watch the wind on Lake Tahoe, as you would on any large lake. Getting caught in rough water is unlikely to be dangerous, because

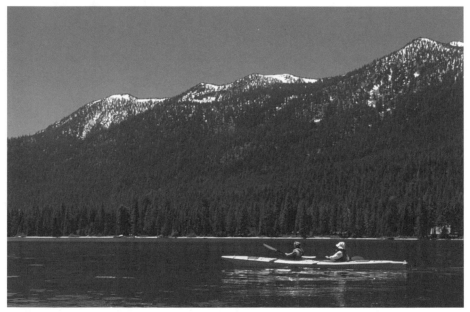

Rubicon Bay on Tahoe's west shore offers good views of the Sierra peaks, and is close to state parks and campgrounds

it is possible to go ashore in most locations. Wind comes up in the afternoon as a rule, so get your paddling done early. If it is windy at daybreak, it will probably be windy all day, so plan not to paddle unless you are experienced and comfortable with conditions.

Cold water is a very real hazard on Tahoe. You won't find bathers languishing in the water for very long at beaches, and the reason is that the water surface temperature varies from 40°F to the mid-60° range. Immersion in water this cold quickly leads to hypothermia and the loss of muscular function. Make every effort to keep your boat upright.

How to Get There

Lake Tahoe is located south of I-80, 32 miles west of Reno, Nevada, and 98 miles east of Sacramento, California. From I-80, turn south on Hwy. 89, 4 miles west of Truckee. Proceed 14 miles south on 89 to the junction at Tahoe City. Turn right (south) at this junction, and continue 10 miles to Meeks Bay. The Forest Service campground is located immediately south of the Meeks Creek bridge.

Area Features, Background, and Tips

The striking granitic mountains around Lake Tahoe owe formation of their light grey rock to molten magma, which rose from deep within the earth but failed to reach the surface. The overlying material then eroded away, exposing the granite that was then subjected to erosion. Sometime between 5 and 10 million years ago, tectonic forces began the western tilt of the Sierra Nevada block of mountains, uplifting the eastern edge. At about the same time, the Carson Range to the east began uplifting and tilting in the opposite direction. The valley in between sank, as the mountains on either side continued to rise along parallel faults. This valley became the site of Lake Tahoe. Though Lake Tahoe did not form from a volcanic caldera, volcanism and ensuing lava flows two million years ago changed stream flows, diverting their waters into the lake. Later, glaciation, which was most active here around 200,000 years ago, shaped the mountains to the west, carving out Emerald Bay and depositing a massive amount of sediment into the lake. Much of this sediment was redistributed by Tahoe currents. No terminal moraines survive, but it was estimated that the glaciers extended as far as a mile into the present lake.

At one time lava blocked the outflow from the lake, causing water levels that were nearly 600 feet higher than those of modern times. But glacial ice carved away the lava dam, leaving the outflow of the Truckee River much as we see it today. Some 63 streams flow into Lake Tahoe, but only one, the Truckee River, flows out, pouring its water east and then north into Pyramid

Lake, a closed system with no outlet to the sea. At present, there is a small dam at Tahoe's outlet, which can control levels by a few feet.

Tahoe was "discovered" in 1844 by Col. John Fremont, guided by Kit Carson, on the same trip that Pyramid Lake was explored. Much has been written of the ill-fated Donner party who wintered near Truckee, a few miles north. The area had a colorful history, being on the routes between San Francisco and the mining territory in Nevada. The railroad conquered the Sierras in 1868, and soon thereafter the resort possibilities of the Lake Tahoe area were recognized.

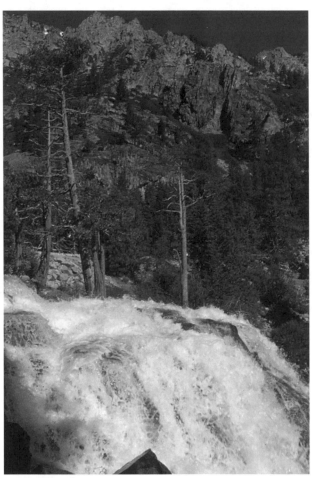

Eagle Creek cascades hundreds of feet into the canyon formed when glaciers carved Emerald Bay

One easy way of travel around the area in early days was by steamship on the lake. Outmoded by 1930, steamboats were retired and newer boats commissioned for the tourist routes. The rising popularity of skiing after World War II was responsible for year-round access to many areas around Tahoe. The Winter Olympics at Squaw Valley in 1960 assured the area a place as one of the great ski areas in the world. With water being the main attraction in summer and ski areas attracting thousands in winter, Lake Tahoe now has a year-round economy, due also in large part to the gaming casinos in Nevada at South Lake Tahoe.

There are five USFS campgrounds around Lake Tahoe, as well as five state campgrounds. The Forest Service campgrounds are operated as concessions by California Land Management, Inc. This trip begins at the Forest Service campground at Meeks Bay. If for some reason it is full or not open, you can investigate the private campground at Meeks Bay Resort, on the north side of the creek. There is a marina in conjunction with this resort, but you can launch from the beach just as easily.

A few of the campgrounds have sites that are near the water, while others are across the roadway from the lake shore. One state park, D. L. Bliss, on the west shore between the lake and the highway, has some sites quite close to the shoreline. The destination of this trip is the Emerald Bay Boat Camp, a state park facility accessible by boat only and located in Emerald Bay. There are toilet facilities, camp tables, and piped drinking water. The 10 sites are available on a first-come, first-served basis. At this writing there is a $9 fee to camp. Use regulations for the boat camp may vary, so check before you go.

Lake Tahoe water is suitable to drink after treating or filtering it, so you needn't carry an excessive amount in your boat. Be sure you take insect repellent, as mosquitoes can be plentiful ashore in the spring and early summer. Respect the pristine nature of where you are, and leave no rubbish or sign of your having been there. To keep Tahoe blue, jet skis have been banned there. Larger boats must use certain specific, non-toxic bottom paints, and other environmental controls are in force.

There are other trip possibilities on Tahoe for the kayaker. Circumnavigating the lake is a 71-mile trip. If the far shore seems a long distance away, it is; Tahoe is 12 miles across and 22 miles in length. Even for a lake of 193 square miles at 6,229 feet in elevation, it's surprising that the average depth is 989 feet, with the deepest spot being 1,645 feet below the surface. No wonder the clear water takes on such a deep, cobalt blue.

Trip Description

From Meeks Bay, paddle south along the west shore. Within 0.5 mile, you will round the southern point enclosing the bay and be paddling in Rubicon

Bay, a shallow indentation some 2.5 miles in length. Near shore, large granite boulders are visible at varying depths. Sand bottom farther out gives the water a green color, until still farther out the characteristic blue of Tahoe water dominates. There are vacation cabins along this section of the lakeshore, which is characterized by steeply sloping, brushy swales, dotted occasionally with conifers. At various places on the hills, you can see granite boulders deposited by glaciers, just as were those below the surface, under your kayak.

At the south end of Rubicon Bay is Rubicon Point (3 miles from launch). Here, shoreside development ceases, for the land is a part of D.L. Bliss State Park. Paddle close to the cliffs at Rubicon Point, and reflect on the more than 1,000 feet of water beneath your boat. You are near the fault line east of which the Tahoe Basin sank along the vertical surfaces of Rubicon Point. Had the glaciers, which carved away at the eastern slopes of the Sierra, not deposited vast amounts of material into the lake, no one knows how deep the water would be at this point.

Continue south 2.5 miles, enjoying the water and the largely pristine shoreline. Some of the state park campsites are close to the water along this section. As you approach the entrance to Emerald Bay, you'll notice that the lake becomes quite shallow. The two low points of land that guard the

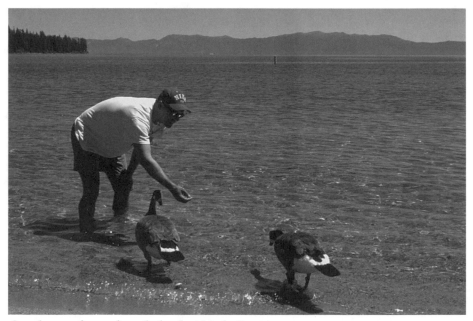

Canada geese forage along the beach at Meeks Bay

entrance on either side project well out into the lake. Sand, gravel, and boulders, left behind when the last glacier gouging out Emerald Bay melted, created a shallow narrows leading into the main lake. Buoys mark the channel here, important for boats with deep draft. In your kayak, you can sneak over the bar at any place where there is sufficient water beneath you (5.5 miles from launch).

Immediately inside the Emerald Bay entrance, paddle in a southwesterly direction. The island 1.5 miles ahead is Fannette Island, a popular spot for boat enthusiasts to visit. Sometimes various tour boats also visit this island. But if you are like many paddlers, the vistas that will enthrall you are of the towering slopes at the head of Emerald Bay. Cascading waterfalls are visible, as Eagle Creek tumbles down granite slabs into the bay. You can easily imagine the steep canyons above filled with glacial ice, slowly forming the bay you are on.

The Emerald Bay Boat Camp is located on the north shore 0.6 mile inside the entrance to Emerald Bay. It is hard to enter Emerald Bay in a kayak and not want to paddle all around it, but secure your campsite before doing so. Being at water level in such a massive, steep-walled canyon is a unique and inspiring experience. To return to Meeks Bay, retrace the route you paddled.

Alternate Trips

While the author has paddled only the trip described in this chapter, it's one of many that are possible at Lake Tahoe. A good way to scout additional lakeshore routes is by car, spotting suitable camping possibilities. These will in every case be some sort of developed camp, as shoreline camping is not allowed on the lake. After you pin down your overnight stops, you can drive back to the beginning and then paddle the route. Fallen Leaf Lake, a short distance south of Hwy. 89 between Emerald Bay and South Lake Tahoe, is a 1-mile-wide, 3-mile-long natural lake of great beauty. There is a marina and a Forest Service campground on Fallen Leaf Lake.

Other Area Activities

Hiking trails abound around Tahoe. One memorable hike begins along Hwy. 89 at the west end of Emerald Bay, and leads up Eagle Creek into the Desolation Wilderness. Parking fees are in effect at the trailhead, and permits must be secured in advance for wilderness entry. Check with the administrative agency.

Several of the ski areas operate lifts and trams during the summer season; some evening trips include dinner. Trails are often accessible at the top of the lifts.

Virginia City, the most famous silver boomtown of the past, is located near Carson City, Nevada. Many other historic attractions are nearby, including the site of the Donner party camp, at Donner Lake near the town of Truckee, just north of Lake Tahoe.

And last but not least, there is the glitz of the casinos and shows at Stateline, on the south shore.

Contacts

For trail information, maps, and regulations:

USDA—Forest Service
Lake Tahoe Basin Management Unit
870 Emerald Bay Road, Suite 1
South Lake Tahoe, CA 96150
(530) 573-2600

Emerald Bay Boat Camp
(530) 525-7277

Meeks Bay USFS Campground
(530) 544-5944

Meeks Bay Resort and Marina
(530) 525-6946

D. L. Bliss State Park
(530) 525-7277

California Campground Reservation System
(800) 444-7275

National Recreation Reservation System
(800) 280-2267

Water sliding beneath our bow is green and getting lighter as we approach the beach, then turn sharply and parallel the shore. Beneath us, 8 feet down, is light beige sand composed of Sierra granite. We can almost see the large, individual grains. Ahead, rising nearly out of the water, is a rounded boulder, causing just the slightest ring on the lightly riffled surface. We change course to miss the rock and at the same time spot a large trout cruising the shallows, looking for minnows that swim there. The trout sees or senses us; quick, powerful tail flicks power the fish to deeper water and out of view.

A short time later, after passing a point on which rounded boulders the size of houses march down and into the water, we paddle along a vertical cliff face. The water beneath the kayak looks like ink, dark blue ink. And a strange thrill runs through us.

Our boat floats over water 1,000 feet deep, not uncommon but still awe-inspiring within yards of the shoreline. Though there is little difference between 1,000 feet and 20 feet in terms of flotation, pondering these watery depths creates an ominous sense of danger.

We enter Emerald Bay in a light chop, keeping to the north shore. Though not our first time here, the powerful aura of the flooded, glacial-carved canyon is formidable. The bay runs west, shallowing on sediments brought down from Eagle Creek. The same creek cascades above over granite ledges, glistening in the sunlight. Mid-bay in the near foreground is Fannette Island, projecting granite cliffs, pine trees, and brushy slopes well up above the water's surface. As if orchestrating the scene, atop the island is a human-made, rock-walled structure. Incongruous amid this natural splendor? Perhaps, but somehow it seems not to matter. The grandeur of the bay and the Sierra backdrop is so much greater.

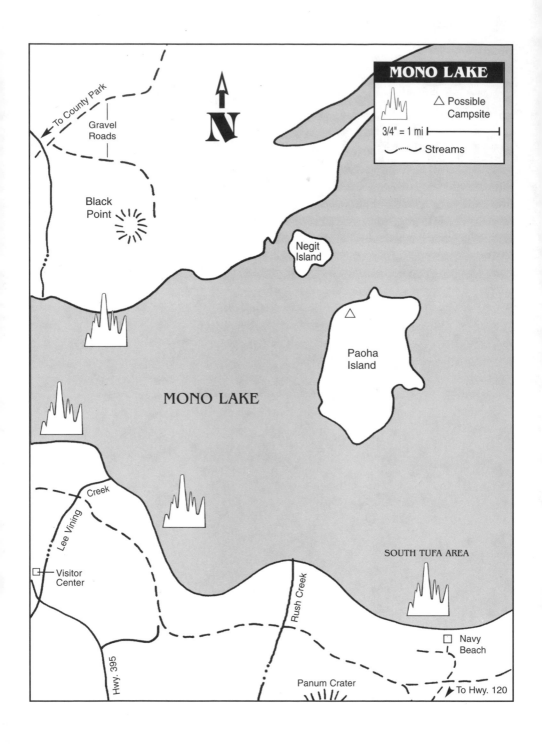

California

Chapter 12

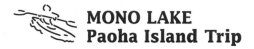 **MONO LAKE**
Paoha Island Trip

Trip Details

Distance:	10 miles (wind permitting) or 14- & 28-mile options
Time:	4-? hours paddling
Rating:	Easy to Moderate
Maps:	USGS 7.5-min: *Negit Island*, *Sulphur Pond*, *Mono Mills*, and *Lee Vining*

Summary and Highlights

Mono may be the most unique body of water you will ever paddle! Just half a dozen miles west of this 60-square-mile lake, the eastern Sierra peaks rise to over 12,000 feet. To the north the silver-producing Bodie Hills amass to 9,000 feet, and when you turn south, you are facing Mono Craters, a volcanic landscape as moonlike as anything you're likely to see. In the center of the lake, Paoha Island is the site of one of the latest volcanic eruptions, around 250 years ago. Your paddle encounters more-than-customary resistance and your kayak rides high; Mono Lake water is 10% mineral.

Dozens of earthquakes each day vibrate the region, and have for the past decade or more. Twenty miles south in the ancient Long Valley caldera, molten magma rising from deep within the earth has uplifted the valley 2 feet since the mid-1980s, a rapid event in geological time. So if you expect to paddle Mono and escape an aura of the unusual, think again.

Aside from the ravishing scenery, from which paddlers can hardly tear their eyes, the bird life makes the next most powerful impression at Mono. About 50,000 California gulls populate a nesting colony on Mono Lake islands. Ornithologists estimate that 90% of the California population of this gull is born at Mono Lake. These gulls are smaller, and less raucous and obnoxious than some of their cousins at the seashore. Up to 100,000 Wilson's phalaropes visit the lake in summer, remaining until early fall before beginning an astonishing migratory flight to South America. Not to be outdone, the eared grebe migration in September and October may bring more than 1 million of these small diving birds to the lake. Feeding on brine shrimp, the grebes have the ability to dive deep, accessing shrimp that other predators cannot reach. There are many other species present seasonally, and as permanent residents.

For a lake more than two times as salty and 80 times as alkaline as sea water—one that Mark Twain called a "dead sea"—Mono Lake probably has a more productive web of life (food chain) than nearly any of its freshwater counterparts. Prominent to this web are two unusual animals: the alkali fly and the brine shrimp. Both reproduce in astronomical numbers in the heavy Mono water, providing sustenance for the multitudes of birds. There are no fish in the lake. Your first glimpse of Mono Lake from the highway also reveals clusters of stonelike columns—called "tufa towers"—rising above the water and from land areas near the shore. You will become more familiar with these formations when you spend time paddling here.

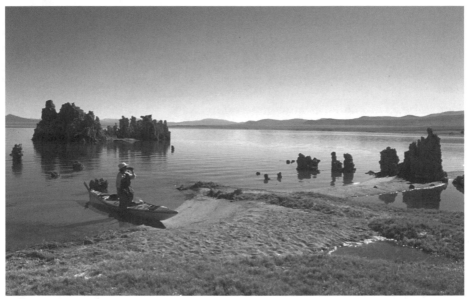

On Mono Lake's south shore this sandspit site has it all—wildlife, tufa formations, and a pleasant beach

On first glance you may evaluate Mono Lake only as a great spot for a day paddle. A day trip there is memorable. But consider that approximately 15 miles of lakeshore offer boat camping without competition from vehicle campers. With the exception of a closure to protect nesting birds, the north half of Paoha Island is also open to camping, providing a very unique experience. Paddle-boat camping on Mono is more than just birds and more birds. Imagine watching the sun slip behind snowcapped Sierra peaks as their shadow races toward you, the birds retreat to roosts, and then the nighttime sky sparkles in a way it can only do at 7,000 feet. The next morning you are awakened early, as sunrise arrives over the low-elevation, eastern horizon. Paddling on Mono Lake is not humdrum.

When to go: This overnight trip schedules camping on Paoha Island. Mono Lake islands are closed to access from April 1 to August 1 each year to protect nesting birds. If your trip falls during the closure dates, you must substitute camping in one of the shoreline areas described later in this chapter.

By May desert shrubs are blooming, as are some wildflowers. The Sierra passes are about to open from winter snow closures, and daytime temperatures can reach into the 70s. Nights are cold, though, in the 20s to low 30s. While spring winds can be very unpredictable and unexpected snowstorms can appear out of nowhere, this is a good time for the hardy paddler. By early summer, willows and cottonwoods are in full leaf and daytime temperatures are in the 80s. Be aware that thunderstorms are common in the afternoon. This is a good time for a trip on the lake. Early fall is also ideal, with cooler days and brisk nights. Winters here are severe, with snow on the ground and all freshwater lakes frozen. Yet its high mineral content usually protects Mono Lake from freezing.

Hazards: Sudden, strong winds are the greatest hazard on Mono Lake. Its location near the high Sierra peaks makes the lake basin subject to strong gravity winds with little or no warning. Both the Forest Service and the Mono Lake Tufa State Reserve personnel warn of their danger to boaters. The admonitions are more than idle talk, and it makes sense to stay close to the lakeshore. By traveling from one side of the lake to the other via the shoreline, you'll be safer and see more. If you are crossing to the islands, it is much safer to access them from the north shore, a route which offers the shortest open-water distance. Unfortunately, watching the distant water surface on Mono Lake provides only a minute or two warning of approaching winds.

Be sure to carry water with you. Whether camping or just day paddling, the arid climate at 7,000' elevation means your body will use more water than usual. You can't just treat or filter the lake water here (as you can on many of the trips in this book), so bring fresh water for rehydration, cooking, and camp chores.

Mosquitoes can be fierce for a short time in the spring after the snow melts. After that, the numbers of these pests diminish. It is a good idea, however, to bring repellent.

The elevation of the Mono Basin is not ideal for reptiles and, as a consequence, rattlesnakes are not numerous here. They are present, however, so use normal precautions.

In early spring and late fall, seasonal cooling lowers water temperatures to levels that will bring on rapid hypothermia to a person who is immersed. The fact that you and your boat float higher in Mono Lake water won't help much, so stay within your capabilities and keep your boat upright.

How to Get There

Mono Lake is on Hwy. 395, directly east of Yosemite National Park, 125 miles south of Reno, Nevada, and 25 miles north of Mammoth Lakes, California.

Area Features, Background, and Tips

The landscape we see today at Mono Lake is still being shaped by both volcanic and tectonic activity. The Sierra Nevada range has been rising continuously, while the eastside valleys have been sinking. This process has been going on for 4 million years, just a wink in geologic time. The lake is thought to be more then 760,000 years old, formed about the same time a cataclysmic volcanic eruption 25 miles to the south hurled 150 cubic miles of molten rock into the atmosphere. The crust sank more than a mile, forming the initial basin. Over time the western edge of the basin has slipped downward, while the north and south portions have tilted toward the center. The resultant tublike depression filled with water is Mono Lake.

After the peak of the last great ice age some 12,000 years ago, Mono Lake rose as vast amounts of ice melted and overflowed the basin for a short time. The eastside Sierra glaciers receded and, gradually, the supply of water from melting ice diminished. Water levels dropped—largely through loss to evaporation. Except for during the ice-age overflow, there has been no outlet for Mono Lake. For three-quarters of a million years, Sierra streams have leached minerals from rocks and washed these compounds into Mono Lake. As the lake water evaporated, these salts were left behind, gradually raising its mineral level. Today, Mono water is 2.5 times saltier than sea water. Total mineral content nears 10% by weight. No wonder your paddle feels solidly anchored in the water here.

But glaciers and water have played only a part. Volcanism is directly responsible for most of the landscape you now see to the north, east, and south of the lake. The Bodie Hills on the north are of volcanic origin, millions of years old. The same is true of the Anchorite Hills to the east. Virtual new-comers, the Mono and Inyo craters south of the lake have been active for the last 40,000 years, erupting and mountain-building every few hundred years. The craters, a series of rhyolitic domes, share the distinction of composing the youngest mountain range in North America. The most recent eruption in this area occurred on Paoha Island, in the middle of the lake, about 250 years ago. Nearby Negit Island has not erupted for 1,700 years. This island area is still active, as evidenced by hot springs and steam vents on Paoha. Scientists think that the next volcanic eruption in the region will occur somewhere along the Mono/Inyo crater chain.

The unusual spires and towers out in the lake are tufa towers. Tufa is a stone material similar to limestone, chemically known as calcium carbonate. The mineral-laden waters of Mono Lake provide the carbonates, while the calcium is supplied by bubbling springs. The formation of calcium carbonate around an upwelling spring is a slow, steady process resulting in a tufa tower. Today you can spot many tufa formations far above the present lake level, just one sign that the lake was much higher in the past. Tufa only forms beneath the surface, where the lake water can supply the carbonates needed for the reaction. Tufa-forming activity can be seen in shallow water a few

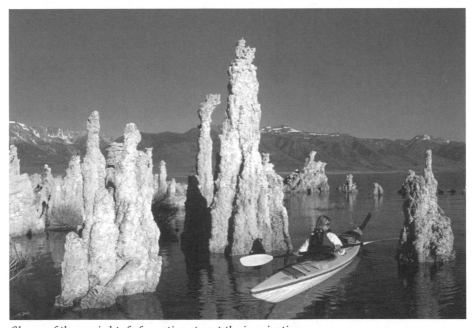

Shapes of the myriad tufa formations taunt the imagination

hundred yards west of the launch area at Navy Beach. Look for gas bubbles noisily breaking the surface.

Sand tufas are another interesting form of the phenomenon. They are also formed underwater, by calcium-bearing freshwater springs percolating upward through briny, sandy lake bottom. Receding lake levels have exposed the sand bottom. Winds blow away the loose sand, exposing intricate columns and tubes of harder sand, cemented by calcium carbonate. Sand tufas are very fragile. Examples may be seen on the south shore near the Navy Beach parking lot.

Black Point, on the north shore opposite Negit Island, was formed by an underwater volcanic eruption that occurred around 13,000 years ago when the lake level was elevated because of ice age melting. The summit area of Black Point cracked as the cold water caused contraction, leaving fissures in the rock. While only a few feet or yards wide, the fissures are as much as 50 feet deep.

On the south shore of Mono Lake, Panum Crater is the result of a much more recent eruption. About 600 years ago, magma rose from deep within the earth's crust and contacted water just below the surface. The water expanded into steam, causing a large, violent eruption that threw out enough material to leave a gaping crater behind. Visitors to the crater can see all of the classic characteristics of a rhyolitic, plug-dome volcano at Panum. The high silica content of Panum lava has resulted in pumice and obsidian formation. The crater is reached off Hwy. 120, 3 miles east of Hwy. 395 south of Lee Vining.

The modern-day newsmaker in the Mono Basin hasn't been volcanic activity; it's been water. The liquid commodity that spawned range wars when the west was developing has been no less emotionally and ruthlessly fought over in present times. In 1941, the Los Angeles Department of Water and Power completed an aqueduct that carried water 350 miles from the Mono Basin to Los Angeles. This was appropriated water for Mono Basin lands, and Los Angeles obtained water rights to it by condemning and then purchasing large tracts of land in key areas of the Mono Basin. The system diverted four of the six streams that previously flowed into Mono Lake. Deprived of this inflow, the lake began to shrink in size because more water evaporated each year than was gained from runoff and precipitation.

Mono Lake shrank to half the volume it had before the diversions took place. The same amount of salts remained, which in effect doubled the lake's salinity. As the shoreline receded, wetland areas shrank and—along with increased salinity—made Mono Lake less usable by the millions of migrating waterfowl that historically were present. The birds' food sources in the lake became less abundant, as the sudden increase in salinity caused water organisms—principally the brine shrimp and the alkali flies—to diminish both in size and numbers. An additional negative impact as lake size diminished was the exposing of large areas of lake bottom. Fine sediments of these alkali flats become airborne when strong winds blow, enough to make the Mono Basin in violation of federal air-quality standards. Negit Island, formerly a haven and rookery for nesting birds, became accessible to the mainland via a peninsula, which was exposed as the water level receded. Gulls and other species were forced to abandon their rookeries there in favor of smaller islets where land predators could not reach their nests.

Many concerned citizens—in the area and throughout the West—became vocal about the issues at Mono Lake. As a result, in 1982 Mono Lake Tufa State Reserve was established to preserve the spectacular tufa formations and other features of Mono Lake. The reserve consists of state-owned lands below the elevation of 6,417 feet, the lake level before the 1941 diversions. In 1984 Congress established the Mono Basin National Forest Scenic Area to protect the cultural, scenic, and natural resources of the area. The great war over water came at the end of lengthy, complicated proceedings in 1994, when the State Water Resources Control Board decided that the management level of Mono Lake will rise 17 feet over the next two decades to an elevation of 6,392 feet. The interested parties with standing in the dispute have agreed to this decision, and have moved forward to implement it. Diversions have been modified, and today the lake level is rising. Mono Lake—for now at least—has been "saved."

It's best to begin your visit to Mono Lake at the Scenic Area Visitor Center, just north of the town of Lee Vining. Here, knowledgeable volunteers and staff can provide information, and you can view an excellent film and other interpretive material about the Mono Basin. This is where you will get your permit to camp on the open areas of Mono Lake shoreline.

Camping is prohibited on Mono Lake's western shore from Black Point south to 2.5 miles east of Navy Beach. In addition, there are spot closures around different springs, and on all Los Angeles Department of Water and Power land on Paoha Island. Secure a large-scale, accurate map, and make sure you check with reserve personnel to locate all closed areas. Pack out everything you take in, including your feces. The Mono Lake ecosystem is far too precious to pollute.

Land and waters within 1 mile of Mono Lake's islands are closed to all entry from April 1 to August 1 each year to protect nesting birds. Not only may you not land on the islands, don't paddle closer than a mile. The whole lake is a good place to showcase responsible paddling ethics. Since just being on the water has impact, it is especially important to avoid harassing the bird life, even unintentionally. Birds moving away from you are an indication you have approached too close.

Of particular interest is the southeastern shore, east of the closed area. There are sandspits, small ponds isolated from the lake by wave-created spits, points covered with salt grass, and lots of interesting features. Gulls and other birds use these areas for resting during the day. Inland a few hundred yards from the present shore, sage brush grows on the gentle slopes. The usual rodent inhabitants are present here, and so is the occasional, restless coyote.

Trip Description

Launch at Navy Beach 5 miles east of U.S. Highway 395 off of Hwy. 120. A sign identifies the gravel road that turns left (north) toward the lakeshore. An old dock at Navy Beach, used when lake levels were much higher, is now far above the water level. Small gravel areas on either side of the old dock make good launching sites at this writing. Get on the water as soon after daylight as possible, to complete your paddling early.

Paoha Island lies just west of north, 2.5 miles distant. If you are early and the lake is dead calm, you can cross this open water cautiously. If you launch later in the day or if wind indications are present, don't try to cross. Instead, paddle west, following the shore north and finally east to Negit Island. Turn south at Negit, following its shore until you can cut across the 0.7 mile of open water separating it from Paoha Island. Reaching Paoha by this route is a 14-mile paddle, a bit much for those not hardened to the effort. An alternative would be to launch at the Old Marina Site, just off Hwy. 395, 2 miles north of the visitor's center. Doing this will shorten the shoreline route by 7 miles, although you may have to carry your boat a short distance at the Old Marina Site.

The best camping areas on Paoha Island are on its shore, in the area directly across from Negit Island. The south half of Paoha is Los Angeles Department of Water and Power land, and is closed to camping. Remember the summer bird-nesting closure on the islands. If the islands are closed, find a campsite which suits you in the open areas in the eastern half of the lake.

Other Area Activities

Five miles south of Lee Vining, Hwy. 158 branches off Hwy. 395 to form the June Lake Loop. There are four lakes accessible on this 15-mile-long loop, and seven campgrounds. Besides offering great day paddles on the lakes, the loop campgrounds might be used as a base for your activities in the area.

To get a real taste of volcanic wastelands visit Mono Craters, accessible by primitive roads. A short walk from Hwy. 120 to the Panum Crater will give you insight into events that happened here.

A short interpretive trail through the South Tufa Area (a fee site) is worthwhile. This is one of the largest tufa tower concentrations on the lake.

At the northwest end of Mono Lake—at the County Park—a boardwalk provides access to several different environments. This is where to go if you are interested in the greatest variety of bird life in the area. A picnic area, with tables, mowed grass, and toilets, is located in the park.

Gravel roads take you to Black Point, east of the County Park. It's a 1-mile walk from the road's end to the top of Black Point, on loose pumice and volcanic sand. Allow an hour to reach the summit, and be sure to take drinking water. Remember that the elevation is nearly 7,000 feet. The fissures are on a portion of the point, below and about one-quarter mile west of the summit's highest point. There is no trail, and walking along the edge of the fissures can be dangerous.

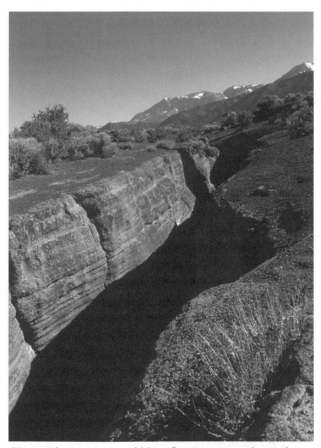

Fissures from centuries-old lava flows are seen today at the top of Black Point

Bodie, a late 1800s and early 1900s mining town 10 miles north of Mono Lake, is reached via a 12-mile drive on a gravel road leading east from Hwy. 395. Since much of this historic town is intact, you can see many buildings and their contents as they were when the inhabitants left. Bodie is now a state park, with visiting hours rigidly controlled to help preserve the artifacts. Access to Bodie is not possible in the winter because of snow in this high-elevation locale.

Contacts

Camping permit, maps, current closures, and regulations:
Mono Basin Scenic Area Visitor Center
PO Box 429
Lee Vining, CA 93541
(619) 647-3044

Mono Basin National Forest Scenic Area
PO Box 429
Lee Vining, CA 93541
(760) 647-3044

Mono Lake Tufa State Reserve
PO Box 90
Lee Vining, CA 93541
(760) 647-6331

Volcanism, facts about Mono/Inyo craters and their current activity:
U.S. Geological Survey
Mail Stop 977, 345 Middlefield Rd.
Menlo Park, CA 94025

The gulls were just returning to feeding grounds near the tufa towers when we slipped our big, double kayak into Mono Lake. After stowing gear, we paddled out onto a surface of burnished silver, where gulls were randomly moving about, dipping beaks below the surface to feed. The growing light from the east was not yet sufficient to see the brine shrimp, which were breakfast for the gulls. The water feels heavy, dense—somehow resistant to the movement of our paddles.

The first rays of sunlight came as we were passing a group of tufa towers. With amazing rapidity their dull gray turned to a tarnished gold. At the same time, the sky above the snowcapped Sierra peaks achieved a deep blue, reflecting at a low angle on the lake surface. Swallows initiated swooping flights from the tufas, plowing through insect concentrations. As the sun cleared the horizon and full light reached the tufas, an osprey pumped by in determined flight, off to freshwater lakes to catch a morning meal. There is a duck out there among the gulls, but too distant for us to identify.

We linger among the gnarled, golden towers of tufa, unable to leave. It is other-worldly, full of shapes that suggest familiar animals or caricatures. And the sky-peak reflection is getting stronger. We take pictures or just sit still in the boat, letting this place sink in.

The realization that time is passing stirs us from our trance, and we extricate our-selves carefully from the tufa maze, careful not to touch the delicate formations. Nearby gulls object vociferously to our presence, and we make a wide detour around the birds. The water teems with brine shrimp, of which the gulls are well aware. Soon we are clear of the birds and steady on our course to Paoha Island.

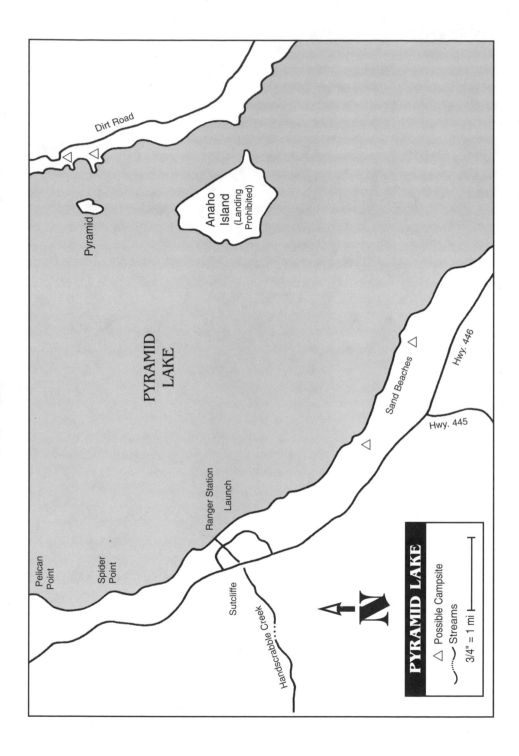

Nevada

Chapter 13

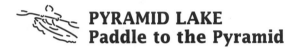

PYRAMID LAKE
Paddle to the Pyramid

Trip Details	
Distance:	10 miles
Time:	5 hours paddling
Rating:	Moderate to Difficult
Maps:	USGS 7.5-min: *Sutcliffe* and *Nixon NW* Also, Map Brochure B70441 (09/93), Pyramid Lake Paiute Tribe

Summary and Highlights

Would you like to paddle around the same towering rock spotted by Captain John Fremont, as he explored Nevada in 1844? "We encamped on the shore opposite a very remarkable rock in the lake, which had attracted our attention for many miles. This striking feature suggested a name for the lake, and I called it Pyramid Lake."

Pyramid Lake, like Mono Lake in California, is the terminus lake in a closed drainage system. The lake is a relic of a much larger, prehistoric lake that covered hundreds of square miles of Nevada desert. The source of water for Pyramid Lake is the Truckee River and its tributaries, including the entire watershed area of Lake Tahoe on the California-Nevada border. All of Pyramid Lake lies within the Pyramid Lake Paiute Tribe Reservation, and is administered by the tribe.

The rating of this trip is "Moderate to Difficult" only because it involves a 5-mile, open-water crossing. Because Pyramid Lake is 26 miles long and from 4 to 11 miles wide, there's plenty of area for winds to build up more-than-respectable wind waves. On a flat day, though, this paddle is a piece of cake.

You can expect to see unusually shaped towers and other tufa features, which are actually calcium carbonate deposits formed by the chemical reaction when calcium in underwater springs combines with carbonates in the lake water. As soon as you launch, the striking pyramid-shaped rock across the lake will draw you toward it. You may wonder how this unusual, towering landmark came to be, and, after paddling around it, you will learn the answer. To camp on the sand-and-gravel shore near the pyramid and watch the sunrise illuminating it is a highly moving experience. A narrow, sandy beach awaits you, while just above is a gravel shelf ideal for camping. Irregular tufa formations create private alcoves just begging you to pitch your tent. Gulls wheel above, and an occasional raven may call mournfully from the desert. It is very easy to imagine Pyramid Lake as it was before Fremont arrived.

This is a high-desert lake. The surface elevation is 3,796 feet, plus or minus a few feet to allow for seasonal and drought-cycle variations. Being the catch basin for a river system with no outlet to the ocean, it is not surprising that Pyramid has a salt content one-sixth that of sea water. While you wouldn't want to drink much of it, the water in Pyramid Lake is apparently just fine for huge cutthroat trout. These famous fish, some of which ran up to 39 lbs. and spawned in the Truckee River, made Pyramid Lake a mecca for trophy anglers. Diversion of Truckee River water in 1903 ended the fishery, which has been restored in recent decades by a concerted tribal effort. Fish are an important part of Paiute culture, for a type of sucker called *cui-ui* that live in the lake were the staple food for this tribe centered around Pyramid Lake. *Cui-ui* were heavily impacted by the water diversion, and have been on the Endangered Species List since 1967.

Paddling on Pyramid is possible year-round. And if conditions are unfavorable for a crossing, there are other trips that can be paddled along the shore. An added feature here is many miles of sandy beaches, all open to camping when you purchase a tribal permit. You will also need a boating permit to launch and use your kayak on the lake. If you fish, you will need a tribal permit, also; Nevada fishing licenses are not valid within the reservation.

When to go: Pyramid Lake does not freeze, and paddling is possible during the winter. However, the elevation plus the east-of-the-Sierra location results in chilly temperatures and downright cold, winter nights. Winter is sunny, except when a storm system is passing through. The Sierras wring most of the moisture from passing clouds. April through early June, and again from mid-September through November, are ideal times to visit, with moderate days and cool nights. Summer is quite warm, with temperatures reaching above 100°F during the day. The fishing season is from October 1 through June 31 at this writing.

Hazards: Wind, with a great big "W." Even a beginner paddler can sense the potential for sudden, strong winds on Pyramid Lake. These can arise without warning, even when the sky is clear. A wind of 30 miles per hour can cause 4' wind waves in some locations. Early morning is the time most likely to be calm, before solar heating warms up the desert and creates thermals, causing air movement. So, getting your paddling done early in the morning is appropriate here.

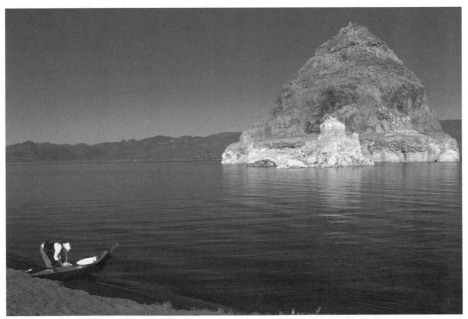

Pyramid Lake's "pyramid" is a massive formation less than a mile from a great camping beach

Be especially wary if thunderstorms are in the area. These cells can form and move quickly, and are usually accompanied by strong winds and sudden gusts. If there is lightning activity, out on the water you offer the highest point around. Go ashore.

Treating lake water is not an option because of the salinity of Pyramid Lake. You will need to carry all of your drinking and camping water with you.

Rattlesnakes are sometimes found on beaches and in the desert. Use caution when camping and going ashore.

How To Get There

From Reno, take I-80 east 30 miles to exit 43 leading to Wadsworth. In Wadsworth, turn north on Hwy. 447. Continue north 16 miles to the junction with Hwy. 446, just south of Nixon. Turn left (west) on Hwy. 446. The Tribal Museum and Visitors Center, an excellent facility and a good source of information, is located on Hwy. 446 near the junction. Drive northwest on 446, 12 miles, to the junction with Hwy. 445. Continue on Hwy. 446 past this junction, 3 miles, to Sutcliffe, the small settlement consisting of a store, ranger station, fueling facility, marina, campground, and launching ramps.

Area Features, Background, and Tips

Nevada is home to what geologists call the "Basin and Range Province," a landscape characterized by a series of tilted fault-block mountains, separated by broad, intervening basins or valleys that have no outlets. Present-day Pyramid Lake occupies the bottom of such a basin, which together with adjoining ones once cradled ancient Lake Lahontan, covering more than 8,600 square miles. Today the Truckee River, originating in the watershed south of Lake Tahoe and flowing through that lake, gathers its various tributaries and eventually winds its way east and north, becoming the source of water in Pyramid Lake. In this undisturbed closed system, there is no way out for Pyramid Lake waters except evaporation.

If Pyramid Lake is a relic of prehistoric Lake Lahontan, so are its creatures. Most famous of these to anglers are the Lahontan cutthroat trout, which are native to the lake and achieve world-record size. These huge trout attracted attention from serious anglers to Pyramid Lake even before the turn of the last century. This was no surprise to the native Paiutes living around the lake, who had utilized the fishery for centuries. While spawning runs of the cutthroat were important for the native people, they were not as highly prized as the endemic species of sucker, *cui-ui*, which was their staple. The local-dialect name for the tribe means *cui-ui* eaters. *Cui-ui* were gathered in the greatest numbers and preserved as food for the winter.

Anaho Island, just off the east shore in the southern third of Pyramid Lake, hosts perhaps the largest rookery of American white pelicans in the West. Just over one square mile in size, Anaho Island is a National Wildlife Refuge. Camping or landing on the island is forbidden.

In 1903, a diversion dam was built on the Truckee River in order to provide irrigation water for the Carson Valley, a large area lying between Reno and Carson City, Nevada. While this water created lush pastures and other agriculture, the diversion dam stopped the spawning run of trout and *cui-ui*. With less water reaching Pyramid Lake, it dropped 80 feet from pre-dam levels to where you see it today. By 1940, the great Lahontan cutthroat trout were extinct in the lake. The *cui-ui* have struggled ever since, and are now given protection by listing as an endangered species.

The 1903 water diversion caused hardship for the Pyramid Lake Paiute Tribe, to whom subsistence fishing was important. Greatly curtailed spawning runs meant few fish, which in turn meant hunger. Water was one apparent key to reestablishing the fish runs. The tribe's political struggle over water allotments lasted for decades. After many years of litigation, allotments beneficial to all competing interests for Truckee River water have been established. With assistance from Nevada Fish and Game and federal agencies, the tribe established a successful fisheries reintroduction and hatchery program, the other necessary element for reviving the fish runs. Tribal hatcheries now manage the lake's fish population, and some of the natural spawning habitat has been restored.

Today, the Pyramid Lake ecosystem is growing healthier. While the Lahontan cutthroat in the lake now are a closely related strain to the originals, the native *cui-ui*, Tahoe sucker, and *tui* chubs are all are doing well. This is important in many ways, not the least of which is the economic well-being of the Pyramid Lake Paiutes. The major income source for the tribe comes from the combined recreational uses of the lake.

When visiting the Pyramid Lake area, remember that you are on the Pyramid Lake Paiute Tribe Reservation. Nevada laws are not in effect here. The tribe is an entity that has the authority to promulgate its own rules, and you—as a visitor—have the responsibility to respect those rules. Regulations affecting most visitor and recreation activities are printed on the back of the map/regulations brochure mentioned at the beginning of this chapter. Be sure to secure this brochure and familiarize yourself with the rules. Failure to do so can result in your inadvertently running afoul of a regulation. The result will be a fine, without recourse for you.

If you remember that permits are needed for camping and boating, and if you make inquiry about any other activities you have in mind, and then buy the necessary permits for the appropriate periods, you will be fine.

Environmental protection laws as well as fish, game, and boating regulations are strictly enforced. At this writing, all permits may be obtained at the tribal ranger station in Sutcliffe.

Trip Description

Launch at the main ramp just south of the store and ranger station in Sutcliffe, on the west shore of Pyramid Lake. There is an area of natural shore beside the surfaced ramp that you can use. If landmarks are not visible across the lake, steer 60° magnetic, which will take you toward the pyramid, passing about 1.5 miles north of the north tip of Anaho Island.

If weather conditions are not favorable, you shouldn't start on this crossing. If you notice signs of increasing wind while you are paddling, use your

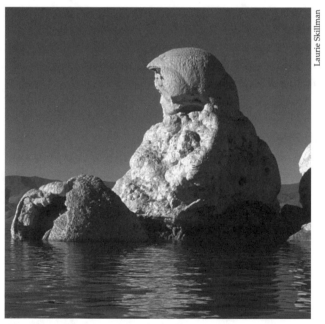

The "Stone Mother and her Basket" bears a striking resemblance from the paddler's perspective

best judgment about heading for the closest shore. While landing is forbidden on Anaho Island, it can certainly be used for a lee shore if things get too sloppy.

Most likely you will be able to see the pyramid across the lake when you start paddling, even though you will be looking into the morning sun. After 3 miles of paddling directly toward the pyramid, you will be at the closest point to Anaho Island. If you paddle during spring or summer, you may be able to see the white pelican rookery on the island. The birds will appear as white flecks, scattered over the gentler terrain of the island.

Continue toward the pyramid, reaching it at 5 miles from launch. As you near the formation, the bulk and height of the landmark are quite impressive. Many paddlers will want to explore around its base. If you do this, keep an eye out for hot mineral springs along the waterline on the south side. Unusual colors from algae and minerals are a clue to the presence of warm springs.

When you're finished exploring the pyramid, continue east a few hundred yards to the beach. The tribe has installed a toilet on the gravel bench above the beach. Just offshore at the south end of this beach are several tufa formations, including the "Stone Mother and her Basket," a formation that apparently has significance for some tribal members. This must be a recent cultural addition, because the formation was under water prior to the early 1900s. There are many camping possibilities on shore in this area. If the presence of the dirt road has attracted other campers to the area, you can consider moving either north or south along the shore to obtain the degree of solitude you desire. Retrace your route to return to the launch point. Be sure to keep an eye out for wind before making the crossing.

Additional Trips

(Note that the author has not paddled these additional routes, but only observed them from land.) If the open-water crossing doesn't appeal to you, or if conditions are unfavorable, you can paddle either north or south from Sutcliffe along the west shore of Pyramid Lake. The west shore has lots of beaches and places to camp. The road follows along the lake the entire way, and some tribal members have their favorite campsites at various locations.

If you wanted to paddle to the pyramid and stay along shore the entire way, the distance is 21 miles via the south shore, one-way from Sutcliffe. As you head north along the east shore from the Truckee River inlet, the roads do not closely approach the shore. Campsites in this area will offer more solitude. Since 21 miles is more than most will want to paddle in one day, this option would make a 4-day, round-trip adventure.

For an even longer trip, the pyramid could be visited from Sutcliffe, paddling via the north end of the lake. The one-way distance is 37 miles. At present, the area around The Needles near the north end of the lake is closed, so be sure to check the current rules. Returning via the south end of the lake would complete a 58-mile circumnavigation of the lake.

Another possibility, if your vehicle is up to it, is to drive north on the dirt road paralleling the east side of the lake. Launch from the east shore, at any spot that suits you, and paddle either north or south along the shore. Be sure to take plenty of water.

Contacts

Pyramid Lake Paiute Tribal Offices
208 Capitol Hill, PO Box 256
Nixon, NV 89424
(702) 574-1000

Pyramid Lake Ranger Station, Sutcliffe
(702) 476-1155

Pyramid Lake Marina, Sutcliffe
(702) 476-1156

The water around us had been flat, but now smooth, oily waves were marching by from the north. As yet there was no wind, but we could see a dark blue line—sign of a confused surface—on the watery horizon. Marching under us were the precursor waves of wind from the north. In the middle of a crossing, paddling harder doesn't help much, but it does make you feel more in control. Luckily, conditions remained stable, and 40 minutes later we slid into the lee of the pyramid.

Until you are paddling within feet of the near-vertical sides of this distinctive landmark, judging its size is difficult. The one thing you are sure of is that it is big. As we explored around the base, we spotted a warm spring venting right at the water line, algae staining calcareous deposits a unique emerald.

Just as interesting as the pyramid, but much smaller in scale, are the tufa formations along shore. We were photographing even before we rounded a rock, and the Stone Mother materialized in front of us. There is little chance of mistaking this distinctive formation. We went ashore to determine if the resemblance remains from that angle, and it does. Somehow the place commands more than a little reverence.

Then it was time for us to head back. We nosed our double kayak away from shore to take a look at conditions to the north; reflecting mill-pond water as far as we could see rewarded us. We set up our even, cruising stroke, and headed west over turquoise-blue water.

Thirty minutes later, a dragonfly landed on the back of Laurie's white hat. I watched it for a minute; the insect was undisturbed and Laurie didn't mind the hitch-hiker, so we paddled on. The excellent conditions held, and just over an hour later we nosed ashore at Sutcliffe. As Laurie was getting out of the boat, the dragonfly flew away, apparently satisfied with the ride but finding us not very significant. Strange, insignificant was what we felt when we were in the middle of Pyramid Lake.

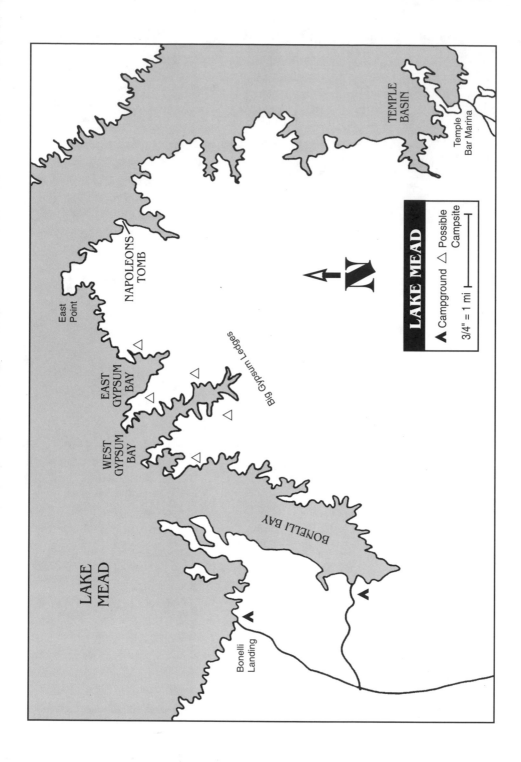

Arizona

Chapter 14

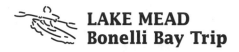 **LAKE MEAD**
Bonelli Bay Trip

Trip Details

Distance:	10 miles (or 18 miles without open-water crossing)
Time:	5 hours paddling
Rating:	Easy to Moderate
Maps:	USGS 7.5-min: *Bonelli Bay*
	NOAA Nautical Chart 18687 (covers the entire lake)

Summary and Highlights

Lake Mead was created when Hoover Dam, a 726'-high structure blocking the Colorado River, was completed in 1935. With a length of 110 miles, the lake is of sufficient size to paddle for weeks and still not see it all. This trip explores a small section of the lake near Temple Bar, about 30 miles downstream (or down-lake) from the western boundary of Grand Canyon National Park. If it were not for the possibility of winds arising, this paddle would be rated "Easy," for it is about as uncomplicated as any trip could be. It is possible to complete this route without any open-water crossings, but doing so will add 8 miles to the total distance. Located in the warm Southwest with an average pool elevation of 1,160 feet above sea level, Mead is not likely to spoil your fun with cold temperatures. The opposite, though, could easily occur. Water temperatures in the 80s are not uncommon during warm months, making swimming a real joy. Mead is a practical and enjoyable, winter paddling destination.

Camping is allowed along most of the shoreline, so paddle trips are easy to plan and even easier to accomplish. Unlike reservoirs that are confined to narrow canyons, Mead inundates gentle topography at full pool and offers moderate slopes for much of the shoreline. This means lots of camping possibilities and practically unlimited bays, inlets, and coves. This trip has as its destination a general camping area rather than a specific campsite. Because there are so many possible campsites in the immediate region, just pick the one that appeals to you. There are literally hundreds of tiny coves—some broad, some as narrow as your boat is long—and many terminate in fine-gravel or sand beaches that make ideal stopping places. However, avoid camping in the bottom of any wash in the event of a thunderstorm with heavy rains.

The contrast from the unimproved camping area where you launch, which is a gently-sloping plain dotted with creosote bushes, to the gypsum cliffs among which you paddle, is marked. You'll see gypsum crystals inches long, scattered about or clustered in great bunches. In places, crystals have formed

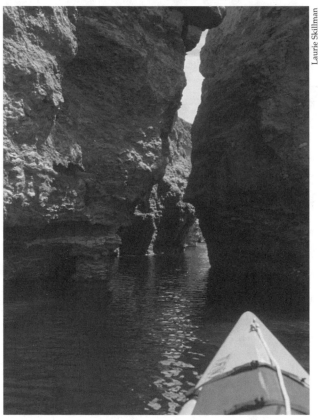

Working your kayak through narrow slots is fun at Lake Mead

columns where waterline conditions are just right. It is a world where sharp angles and low cliffs contrast with extended shallows and gently sloping shores. In short, it is a friendly place to paddle.

When to go: Anytime is appropriate to kayak on Lake Mead. While the coolest months are December and January, paddling is feasible during the winter in the sun-drenched desert. Temperatures at night occasionally reach but rarely dip below freezing, while daytime temperatures average in the 60s. Of more importance to most paddlers is the summer heat. From May through September the temperature can be 100°F or higher. During July and August 110-115° is not uncommon. Unless you like extreme hot weather, avoid paddling Mead during the summer.

Hazards: Wind is the thing to watch out for on Lake Mead. As on all bodies of water—especially large ones—any prolonged wind over 15 miles per hour can cause large wind waves to build. If the fetch is great, such waves can readily exceed the comfort or experience level of paddlers. So watch the distant water horizon for signs of wind—such as a darkening of the surface or, in worse cases, darkening capped by white. Paddle for the nearest shelter in the latter case.

Because of severe heating during the day, spring, summer, and fall thunderstorms are common on Lake Mead. Moisture and slightly cooler air, moving along the monsoon track from the Gulf of California, pass over the area and provide the ingredients for these storms. Such storms can build up rapidly, so the paddler should check the sky frequently for approaching storms. There are two hazards posed by thunderstorms: lightning and wind. When sitting in your kayak out on the water, you are the highest point around. If lightning activity is occurring within 2 or 3 miles, get off the water.

Thunderstorms are accompanied by sudden, strong winds. These can come up without warning, with enough force to capsize your boat. There is a wind phenomenon called "downburst" associated with thunderstorms. Downbursts occur without warning and can reach velocities in excess of 100 miles per hour. It is prudent to get off the water if Lake Mead thunderstorms approach. The National Park Service provides wind-warning "Wind Talkers" at various locations. (Phone numbers are listed under Contacts at the end of this chapter.) There may also be flashing, wind-warning lights at marina locations.

A more insidious hazard is dehydration. In the hot, dry air, perspiration and aspiration can rapidly deplete body fluids, even before you feel thirsty. Be sure to carry and drink lots of water whether or not you feel thirsty. Be aware of the symptoms of heat exhaustion and heat stroke, and the field management of these conditions. Make sure you are protected from the sun by an adequate hat, sunscreen, and glasses.

When camping ashore, remember that rattlesnakes are present. There is also a single species of scorpion that is poisonous. These are small and straw-colored; it's a good idea to shake out your clothing or footgear if it has been lying on the ground.

How to Get There

From Las Vegas, take Hwy. 93/95 southeast for 20 miles to the junction where Hwy. 93 turns east. Turn left (east) on 93 and drive 10 miles to Hoover Dam. A new visitor center is located here. Cross over the dam on Hwy. 93, and continue southeast 19 miles to the junction with a paved, two-lane road that heads north. This road is signed TEMPLE BAR. Turn left (north) and drive 12 miles down Detrital Wash to a junction where the Temple Bar paved road turns 90° East, and a gravel road continues north to Bonelli Bay. Take this gravel road and continue north 4 miles. Here, a fork leads east to Bonelli Bay. Continue north past this fork, and in 2 miles you will reach the end of the road at Bonelli Landing.

Area Features, Background, and Tips

Approximately 24 miles upstream from the head of Lake Mead, the red-rock formations of the Colorado Plateau rise sharply upward in their westernmost battlements. The Grand Canyon is just a short distance from Lake Mead and the spectacular formations exposed there are repeated in lower, gentler profiles throughout the Lake Mead area. The Colorado Plateau landscape is partly uplifted remnants of a 250 million-year-old seabed, and windborne sand accumulations. Other portions are volcanic.

For 11 million years—the time the Colorado Plateau has been uplifting—the Colorado River has been scouring it down. Unbelievable amounts of earth, sand, and rock have been transported along the Colorado River bed—now deep beneath Lake Mead—and out into the Gulf of California. Imagine the top 500 feet of an area half the size of California rasping by, carried by the inexorable river. Such volumes are hard to grasp.

The land area now beneath the lake is much lower in elevation than upstream sites in the Grand Canyon or in Glen Canyon, and as such probably was a favored wintering site for the hunter-gatherer tribes of early peoples who lived in the region. About 1,800 years ago, agriculture began supplementing nomadic foraging; little by little, groups of people living in the region settled down and raised much of their food in one location. These settlements were largely upstream, where greater elevation offered more tolerable summer temperatures. (For more on the geology and history of the Colorado Plateau, see Chapter 15.)

Steamboats powered up the Colorado River from its mouth to the now-long-inundated Mormon settlement of Callville. If you stop at the new visitor center at Hoover Dam, look down at the Colorado River some 726 feet below. Try to imagine steamboat captains pulling their boats upstream through Black Canyon rapids with winches and cables, fighting their way against the current with supplies for mines located in the area. By 1900 the mining activity was diminishing, and the cargo and passenger vessels became a thing of the past. Three decades later, engineers designed a project that would change the desert forever.

Hoover Dam was completed in 1935 after five years' construction. At the time it was the highest dam ever built, and behind it backed up 110-mile-long Lake Mead. While the huge lake altered the ecosystem to the water's edge, a few feet above that border the desert conditions remained as before. Ducks swim on the lake, while a few feet away lizards bake in the sun and rocks heat to temperatures uncomfortable to the touch. Creosote bushes carpet the desert with their evenly spaced patterns. Such are the limited effects of human creations here.

The major impact at Lake Mead is the influx of recreation-minded people. While most come as boaters, skiers, swimmers, sunbathers, or anglers, others come as sightseers, and some to hike and photograph. The Lake Mead National Recreation Area, straddling the Arizona-Nevada border, is more than twice as large as Rhode Island. One of the nicest things about paddling

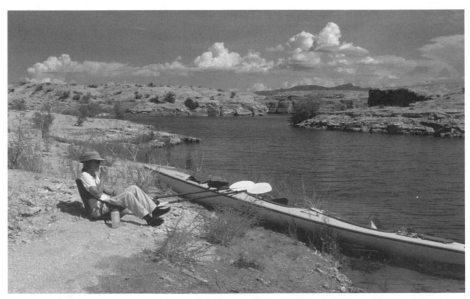

A sunshade would be handy at this lunch spot at East Gypsum Bay

on Mead is the abundance of campsites. If one site does not suit you, paddle on; another possibility will be nearby. If a houseboat or camp occupies a particular cove, simply paddle on until you find another. In spite of the numbers of recreational users, the lake is large enough that you can get away from the hectic activity. The heaviest usage is centered around the major marinas. The Bonelli Bay trip utilizes one of the few access points that is not also the site of a marina.

Boat camping on Lake Mead, in any season requires a sunshade in order to be both safe and comfortable. Shades can be as simple as a light tarp held aloft on one side by two paddles. Vegetation along the shoreline is sparse and usually limited to a few brushy plants, so don't expect to find shade from trees.

You can use the lake water, provided it is either chemically treated, boiled, or filtered. Remember that the lake water will be quite warm, often above 80° in warmer months. If you wish to cool it or other beverages, place tight containers inside a mesh bag with a rope attached, and sink them in deep water. An hour or so submerged will lower the temperature substantially. Use care when retrieving from your aqueous cooler, because the containers will be wet with untreated water. Dry them, remove the lids carefully, then wipe with an anti-bacterial towel.

There are Park Service campgrounds at Boulder Beach, Las Vegas Wash, Callville Bay, Echo Bay, and Temple Bar, the major access points on Lake Mead. Camping is allowed at some unimproved, designated, road-accessible points as well.

Besides the nautical chart for navigation, Park Service offices at Temple Bar (and elsewhere around Mead) sell a cove-name map for the entire recreation area. This map makes it easy to locate coves on Lake Mead that have formal (or recognized) names.

Trip Description

Bonelli Landing is located on a gradually sloping shore dotted with creosote bushes. Several areas have been cleared for primitive camping. There is a pit toilet but no other facilities. Launch by carrying your boat across a rocky shore area to the water—a few yards or many—depending upon lake level.

If you visit during a particularly windy period (if the waves are hitting the shore from the north), you may want to launch instead at Bonelli Bay. The Bonelli Bay launch site is protected by being in a small cove, opening to the somewhat protected waters of the bay itself. But camping is very limited at this launch site. Do not camp in the inviting flat area at the bottom of the wash; it is the drainage point for a 30-mile-long valley south of you.

From Bonelli Landing, paddle east 1 mile, to a rounded cove where the shoreline turns north. Then paddle north for 0.7 mile. At this point, a quarter-mile-long island lies to the west, 400 yards distant. Just ahead, a narrow opening may let you pass eastward, depending upon water level. Here is an intriguing inlet, 800 yards or so across, nestled in the center of the peninsula (at full pool this inlet doesn't exist, just a few islands emerge around the edge). It is a very interesting place to paddle and photograph.

From the inlet entrance, paddle north 0.7 mile, to the north tip of the peninsula (2.4 miles from launch). The area you just passed and the end portion of the peninsula are designated on your chart as the Detrital Reefs. Turn east around the end of the peninsula and, if the wind isn't blowing, make the 1-mile crossing to West Gypsum Bay. (If the wind is blowing too hard for comfort, turn south into Bonelli Bay and follow it around to West Gypsum Bay, adding 8 miles to the paddle.) Just southwest of the west entrance to West Gypsum Bay is an unnamed bay, about 0.5 mile deep, with dozens of mini-coves and inlets to explore. The water in some shoal areas here appears light emerald green above the gypsum bottom.

West Gypsum Bay itself is 2.5 miles long (depending upon water level) and offers dozens of branches, each further broken into myriad tiny coves and inlets, which resulted when this eroded landform was inundated. There are many campsites, so take your pick. Within this bay the water is sheltered if strong winds arise and, if you pick your campsite carefully, your tent will be also. Not too surprisingly, this bay got its name from the extensive gypsum deposits here. You will find striking formations of gypsum crystals and columns in various locations here, as well as along the abrupt western shoreline of Bonelli Bay itself.

East Gypsum Bay, adjoining to the east, is a broader indentation just over 1 mile long. It is striking because of the gypsum formations along its west shore. The east shore is broken by the usual, irregular coves and inlets. Since there is no fixed destination for this trip except West and East Gypsum bays, the trip ends here. Return to the starting point the way you came, or keep to the south (left) shoreline and explore Bonelli Bay on your way back.

Alternate or Additional Trips

(Note that the author hasn't paddled the following routes but has observed them at a distance from shore.) From the turnaround point on the Bonelli Bay trip, paddle east to East Point (2 miles), then continue southeast to Napoleons Tomb and Grebe Bay (2 more miles). All along the south shore in this section are coves and inlets that offer exploration opportunities, and also protection if the wind comes up. Note that winds from northerly directions can have a fetch of several miles along this section.

Another trip possibility from Bonelli Landing is to paddle northwest 6 miles along the shore of Virgin Basin to the entrance of Boulder Canyon. The shoreline is indented with coves the entire way, and some of them will offer shelter. Boulder Canyon, about 5 miles in length, is a narrow constriction in the middle of Lake Mead, with much the same appearance in its narrowest section as the river itself, before it was inundated. Keep in mind that narrow canyons funnel winds that are only breezes on the open lake to greatly increased velocities.

Yet another trip could commence at the marina at Temple Bar and lead east approximately 7 miles to Virgin Canyon, another very narrow section of the lake. While the south shore of this stretch has a number of inlets, winds are more common here than in some of the more open sections of the lake. A paddler would need to select times to paddle, and be prepared to get off the water if doing so seemed advisable.

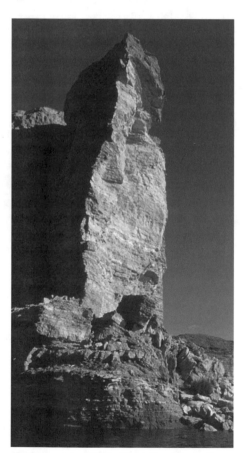

Early morning light silhouettes a formation on Mead's south shore north of Temple Bar

Still another 6-mile paddle might begin at South Cove, the easternmost access to Lake Mead and only a few miles from Grand Canyon National Park, and lead eastward into Iceberg Canyon, the last of three narrows in Lake Mead. Campsites are much less numerous in this section of the lake.

Within Lake Mead National Recreation Area is 67-mile-long Lake Mojave, immediately downstream from Hoover Dam. Much of this lake is very narrow and riverlike. A lazy current exists here, and raft trips are popular from Hoover Dam to Willow Beach, 10 miles downstream. Three paved access roads reach the lake along its length.

Other Area Activities

Hiking in the Lake Mead area offers opportunities to see things that vehicular travelers miss.

Check out the formations near Redstone Picnic Area on the Northshore Road. Rangers can direct you to areas where you can see petroglyphs, old mines, and other things of interest. The best hiking time is from October to May. Make certain you are experienced and equipped for desert hiking. Carry your water, and because the strain of hiking will dehydrate you rapidly, drink frequently.

Contacts
Lake Mead National Recreation Area
601 Nevada Hwy.
Boulder City, NV 89005-2426
(702) 293-8906

Wind and Weather on the lake:
Echo Bay (702) 394-4440

It was like paddling in a bathtub, except that the water stretched for miles in three directions. Glassy smooth water, 84° warm, floated us like a leaf in a pool as we moved slowly along shore. It wasn't the threat of waves or weather that had us following the beach, it was the sparkle of thousands of crystals that attracted us. We saw the reflection of sunlight from the column half a mile away; now the formation was beside our bow, and unlike anything we had seen while boating. Thousands of crystals, each the size of your finger, clustered into a 6'-tall colonnade, rising from below the water to support a gypsum-laden overhang.

Nor was this a single, isolated phenomenon. As we moved along the shore taking pictures, more crystal formations came into view, each with a unique shape. Even the mud at waterline was studded with sparkling crystals.

Later, nearly out of film, we explored the cliff-lined shore of an inlet. Paddling beneath rock overhangs became commonplace, so we negotiated flooded fissures so narrow we had to hand the boat along. Deeper coves sparkled blue; others took on that greenish white that reveals a light-reflecting bottom a dozen or so feet down.

Late morning and still no wind. But we won't push it—won't stretch our luck. The temperature is already over 100°, and rising. It will be nice to stretch out under our sunshade and maybe take a swim. We turn, and head the kayak toward our beach camp.

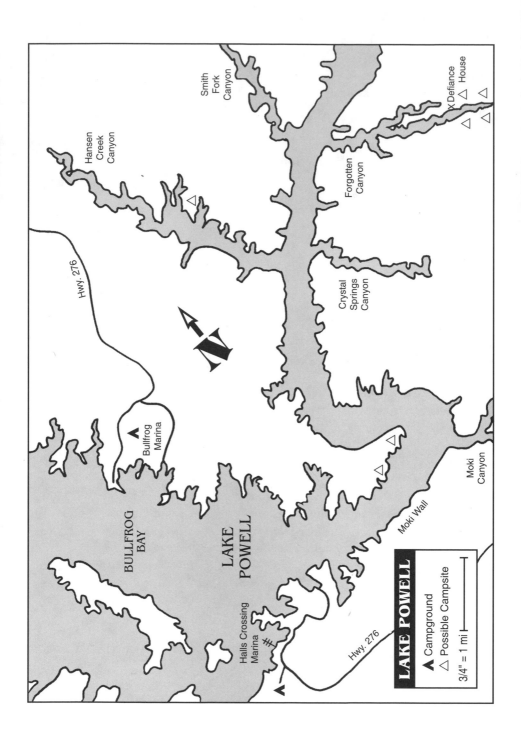

Utah

Chapter 15

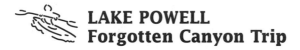 **LAKE POWELL**
Forgotten Canyon Trip

Trip Details

Distance: 26 miles (Moki Canyon side trip adds 9 miles)

Time: 14 hours paddling (4 hours more for Moki Canyon side trip)

Rating: Easy to Moderate

Maps: USGS 7.5-min: *Halls Crossing*, *Bullfrog*, and *Knowles Canyon*

Summary and Highlights

If you've ever wanted to paddle in the red-rock country, Lake Powell is the place to do it. Vertical cliffs of red sandstone form much of the shoreline. You will see river-cut cliffs rising hundreds of feet from the water, some stained with desert varnish and others exhibiting the raw wounds of recent spalling. Overhanging alcoves will shade your boat and lend your voice a theatrical echo.

Lake Powell is big. You can paddle for weeks and not see anything twice. The lake—or more properly reservoir—occupies the area once known as Glen Canyon, a Colorado River canyon located 20 miles upstream from Grand Canyon National Park. When Glen Canyon Dam began backing up Colorado River water in 1963, narrow Glen Canyon was slowly inundated. Side canyons and tributary-cut gulches became inlets of the main lake. The result is a lake 200 miles long, with 1,960 shoreline miles to be explored.

The past is present on Lake Powell even today. Ruins of stone villages, granaries, and steps cut into the sandstone are there if you take the time to seek them out. These are mostly 800-year-old remnants of habitation by Ancestral Puebloans (aka Anasazi). A highlight of this Forgotten Canyon trip is the opportunity to visit Defiance House, a very accessible ruin. The sharp-eyed paddler may also spot stone steps cut into canyon walls at various locations on this trip. When paddling on Powell, think of the canyon you don't see, the one beneath you. Alcoves identifiable at the water line extend below the surface, many of which once sheltered villages. These river-bottom oases succored cottonwoods and rich silt nourished corn and squash, staple crops of the Ancestral Puebloans. Dozens of village sites and untold thousands of artifacts were effectively forever lost, when Lake Powell filled. As you paddle, consider what life may have been like beneath you, at the bottom of Glen Canyon, one millennium ago. At the Defiance House site is also a well-preserved pictograph dating to the same period as the ruins. On the sandstone wall far above reach are painted figures that some think represent three warriors with weapons and shields. Their bigger-than-life stance gives Defiance House its name.

Glen Canyon was named by John Wesley Powell, who explored the Colorado River in 1869. The present lake was named in his honor. His two expeditions—the later one in 1871—explored 1,000 miles of the Green and Colorado rivers, using wooden rowboats. His mapping provided data about the last, great uncharted area within the 48 contiguous United States. Powell later became the head of the United States Geological Survey.

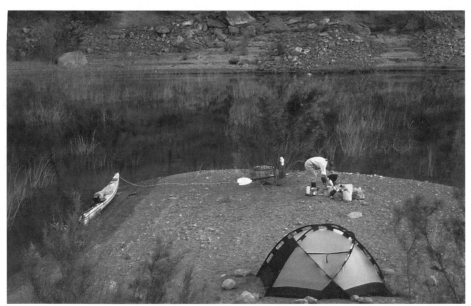

An ideal Lake Powell camp, providing a beach, some shade, and a view, found near The Rincon

Of course the trip to Forgotten Canyon described here is just one of *many* trips possible on Powell. Later in this chapter you will find suggestions for alternate access to the lake, and trips to alternate destinations that Laurie and I have paddled. Forgotten Canyon can be reached in a single day's paddle by most kayakers, and the route is representative of the type of scenery generally offered on this lake.

When to go: Selecting a time to adventure paddle on Powell is an exercise in weighing factors that will affect your enjoyment. The elevation of 3,700 feet above sea level means that winters here can be cold, with a corresponding drop in water temperature. Hot summer temperatures often exceed 100°F with water temperatures that may reach into the 70s. Other boating uses of the lake merit thinking about also. During the summer, recreational powerboat and houseboat usage of the lake is high. The low point of such usage is, of course, during winter. With these factors in mind, perhaps the better times to paddle on Powell are March through May, and late September through early November. While seasonal weather variations do occur, of course, April and October are very good bets for enjoying reasonable weather, and paddling without too much competition from powerboats.

Hazards: It should be no surprise that wind and wind waves are the greatest hazard to paddle boats on Lake Powell. Its sheer expanse of surface area allows wind waves to build. A mile or two of fetch is enough for dangerous waves to occur if wind velocity is above 20 knots. Whenever possible, do your paddling in the morning and save the afternoon, when winds are likely to spring up, for exploring around your campsite or paddling very narrow, protected inlet arms. With strong winds often accompanying thunderstorms, seek shelter if you see an approaching storm, even if there is little wind at the time. In a sheltered spot you will be safer from lightning than out on the water in your boat.

Wakes from other boats are a greater annoyance on Lake Powell than on many water bodies. This is because waves rebound from steep shorelines, and can travel back and forth across an inlet several times before the wave energy is dissipated. Much of the Powell shoreline is vertical cliffs. When several wakes are rebounding in the same vicinity, a real "potato patch" can ensue. Add some wind, and the unsettled, plunging water can become nasty.

For safety sake assume that any fast approaching boat doesn't see you. The majority of powerboat operators are cautious and courteous, but there are unfortunate exceptions. Be ready to wave your paddle overhead in the rare possibility of a boat heading directly for you. Operators with questionable judgment are most likely to be encountered on Lake Powell during the summer.

The geographic location of Lake Powell guarantees direct sunlight in the summer and, even given the elevation, the sun can be brutal. If you paddle during hot weather, protect yourself from burning rays with sunscreen, dark glasses, and clothes to minimize exposure. Camp early in the day to avoid paddling during the hottest time. Take a lightweight tarp to fashion a sunshade in case you are camping on a beach or slickrock. Shady campsites are a rare on Powell. Help to avoid problems by being aware of heat-exhaustion and sunstroke causes and symptoms.

While most campsites on Powell lack enough rodent prey to attract rattlesnakes, use care when exploring brushy ravines or amphitheaters at inlet heads where there is sufficient vegetation for small rodents.

You can use lake water for drinking after filtering, boiling, or chemically treating it. Some of the side canyons have small streams or spring flows, but the quality of these is likely to be no better than the lake water.

How to Get There

From I-40 at Flagstaff, Arizona, turn north on Hwy. 89 and drive 67 miles to the junction with Hwy. 160. Turn right (east) on 160, and drive 82 miles to the junction with Hwy. 163 at Kayenta. Turn left (north) onto 163, and go 42 miles to Mexican Hat. Four miles north of Mexican Hat, turn left (north) onto Hwy. 261. Continue 33 miles to the intersection with Hwy. 95. This segment takes you up onto Cedar Mesa via a short section of gravel switchbacks that offer imposing views of Monument Valley to the south and west. Turn left onto Hwy. 95, and drive 9 miles to the junction with Hwy. 276. Turn left (west) on 276 and proceed 42 miles to Halls Crossing, the put-in point for this trip. (Hwy. 276 continues north of Lake Powell, via a ferry running between Halls Crossing and Bullfrog Marina. Crossing hours vary seasonally, from 8:00 a.m. to sometime in mid-afternoon. Passenger auto fare is $9.)

If approaching from Utah, take the Hwy. 24 loop from I-40—either 8 miles west of Salina, or 9 miles west of Green River. The Hwy. 24 loop goes south to Hwy. 95 at Hanksville. Turn south on 95 and go 26 miles to the junction with Hwy. 276. Turn right (southwest) on 276 and drive 46 miles to Bullfrog Marina. You may then opt to begin your paddle there, or take the ferry across to Halls Crossing.

Area Features, Background, and Tips

The impressive red rocks you see at Lake Powell formed under an extensive, shallow inland sea with fluctuating water levels over a period of over 250 million years. Some of the layers were formed underwater, while others were wind-borne dunes. Uplifting of these stratified deposits some 11 million years ago formed the Colorado Plateau, which stretches from western

Colorado through western Utah, and includes the Grand Canyon in Arizona. The Colorado River, along with its major tributaries, the San Juan and Green rivers, slowly eroded away the plateau surface. Following paths of least resistance, these rivers carved the Canyonlands near Moab, Glen Canyon and—just a few miles downstream—the Grand Canyon itself. Most of the red-rock country is composed of tortured, gouged remnants of the former plateau, eroded away by the Colorado River or its tributary streams.

To grasp the concept of such massive erosion, try to imagine *what isn't there*. When you see a butte or mesa standing in a valley or on an apparent plain, look into the distance to find a similar butte or mesa, with similar rock

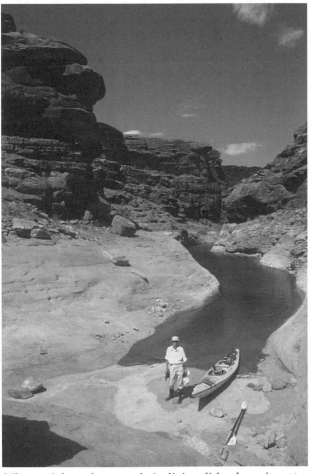

When an inlet ends on gently inclining slickrock, you've got a swimming site if not a campsite, too

strata. Sometimes a matching feature will be miles—or dozens of miles—distant. Then imagine how much rock strata would be required to extend from one feature to another, as it almost certainly once did. Now you have some idea of *what isn't there*. The missing material, hundreds or thousands of cubic miles, was carried away by erosion into the Gulf of California by the Colorado River.

The erosion process includes more than river current wearing away rock. Once the river had cut vertical troughs into the sandstone, other forces began wearing away at the surface. Wind sculpted softer areas, and wore away at harder spots using windblown sand as an abrasive. Water, from rainfall or even dew, seeped into tiny cracks, froze, and—in the expansion of turning into ice—broke off pieces of the surface. The same forces operated more slowly on horizontal surfaces. Sometimes lower portions of the canyon walls eroded faster, creating overhangs, alcoves, or amphitheaters. Forces within the rock caused spalling: the breaking away of thin layers of vertical walls. Where this process progressed from each side of a stone wall, an arch was often formed. Debris from cliffs accumulated at a steep angle at their bases. High water carried away this debris, leaving the lower cliff walls again vulnerable to the erosion process. In this way canyons widen. Surface debris is carried away by winds, or washed away by torrential rains from thunderstorms. Above the surface of Lake Powell, the erosion process is still going on.

By the end of the last ice age, the landscape around Glen Canyon was much as you see it today. Small bands of prehistoric Indians roamed through the canyons beginning around 10,000 years ago. Initially, this was a culture of hunters and gatherers. Agriculture became the base for a new culture around 200 B.C., when corn was domesticated. As corn production increased, the Ancestral Puebloans (Anasazi) gradually established permanent settlements. No longer forced to move to their food supplies, these people dug pit houses into the ground. They were skilled basketmakers, and created functional as well as artistic, decorated pottery.

Was the transition to constructing ingenious and intricate cliff dwellings a natural response to available building materials? Or maybe these pueblos perched on cliffs were a response to enemy raids. Some are constructed so that you have to crawl through a narrow doorway in massive stone works blocking a narrow cliff ledge in order to gain entry. No enemy could breach defenses like that.

Speculation among archaeologists about the sudden departure of the Anasazi focuses on: possible hostility from marauding tribes, extended drought, depletion of soil or degradation of water tables because of stream downcutting, reaching the population maximum, or disease. Whatever the reason, by the late 13th Century the Anasazi were gone from their cliff houses and canyons. The Paiute, Ute, and Navajo tribes gradually succeeded them on the Colorado Plateau; their descendants live there today.

The first documented journey through the area was by two Spanish priests, Dominguez and Escalante. Today the Escalante River, a tributary joining the Colorado near the middle of Lake Powell, bears the name of one of these explorers who were looking for an overland route to California. The Escalante drainage system has been designated a Wilderness Area, one of our newest.

Major John Wesley Powell carried out the first of his two expeditions on the Colorado River in 1869, and the second two years later. Also in 1871, John Lee, acting for the Mormon Church, established a ferryboat service across the Colorado near the south end of Glen Canyon. Pioneers, many of them Mormons from the farming valleys of central Utah, began to move into and settle the area as far south as northern Arizona. Gold was discovered in Glen Canyon in 1871. Flour gold from sand and silt of the Colorado and San Juan rivers was sought first by individual miners and later by organized companies. Various schemes to extract the gold were tried, but dredging and sluicing failed. Mining in the Glen Canyon area faded until the uranium boom in the 1940s and 50s. Then, that too faded away.

By the 1940s, commercial float trips on the Colorado and San Juan rivers were operating, a baby industry from which today's rafting mania evolved. One trip was via airboat from Lees Ferry upstream to visit Rainbow Bridge. Completion of Glen Canyon Dam in 1963 ended float trips on that section of the river, and marked the beginning of recreational use of the huge reservoir that is Lake Powell. In 1972, Congress established Glen Canyon National Recreation Area on more than one million acres surrounding the lake. The area is one of 19 such recreation areas managed by the National Park Service.

The recreation area is open year-round. It is a use-fee area, with entrance permits costing $5 per vehicle for seven days, or $15 annually. There are campgrounds at Wahweap (near the dam), Bullfrog, Halls Crossing, and Lees Ferry. Camping is allowed along the shoreline, making this a great lake for an extensive paddle. To aid in proper sanitation, the Park Service has installed floating toilets and holding-tank pump-out stations at various locations on the lake. Be sure to carry out all your garbage, and deposit feces in the toilets.

Hiking—usually from camps made at the head of inlets—will give you a glimpse of what the canyon bottoms were like before the lake was filled. Walking along sandy washes—whether dry at the time, or harboring a vernal or permanent stream—lets you experience the streamside community of plants at Lake Powell. Even when washes are dry there may be water beneath the sand. Plants growing here are able to tolerate occasional severe flooding as well as periods of drought. The tall trees that grow only near water are Fremont cottonwoods, native to Arizona.

An interesting community of plants make up the hanging gardens. You will see examples of this phenomenon each time you paddle by a cliff or alcove where water is seeping from the rock. Expect to find Gambel oak, maidenhair fern, monkey flower, and possibly columbine. If you hike up streams or washes and encounter a large amphitheater, you may see fantastic displays of hanging-garden flowers in the spring.

Wildlife in Glen Canyon reflects the harsh realities of making a living in country where so much of the surface area is bare rock. Ground squirrels and other small rodents are the most numerous mammals, with the 13 species of bats that live here following a close second. You will see bats after sundown, when they emerge from their daytime sleep in rocky cracks and crevices to catch flying insects. Ungulates (hoofed animals) are represented by the mule deer and the desert bighorn sheep. Neither are particularly numerous, although the sheep population has been reinforced by transplanted herds. Coyotes, foxes, bobcats, and mountain lions are present where their prey species are numerous. It is unlikely you will see any of these predators, although it is not uncommon to hear coyotes yipping at night.

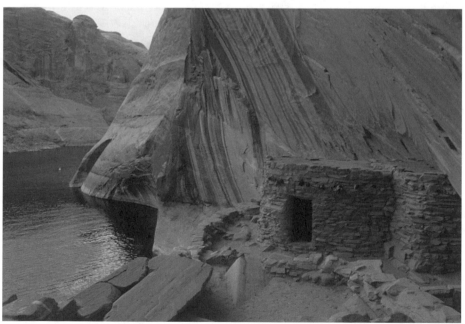

The ruins at Defiance House instill a feeling of reverence in the paddler, who has expended energy to reach Forgotten Canyon

You may see beavers or sign of their workings. Look in areas where willows or cottonwoods grow, at the entry point of streams and washes into inlets. Signs of beaver activity include freshly cut sticks bearing telltale cut marks of teeth, or sticks that have had the bark removed. Sometimes you will spot marks where beavers have dragged limbs across sand or mud into the water. While beavers are mostly nocturnal, they occasionally become active between sunset and full dark.

Several of the more than 200 bird species seen at Lake Powell are especially exciting to spot. Peregrine falcons nest around the lake, which means that you might see one. The peregrine is probably the fastest-flying raptor. Golden eagles seek rodent prey in the areas around the lake during all seasons of the year. Bald eagles visit the area during the winter, looking for fish prey. An unexpected transplant may thrill you at Powell. California condors have been recently reintroduced to the region, and are occasionally spotted. Seeing one of these rare birds, soaring on a wingspan that can reach 9 feet, is an unforgettable experience. Humans have spent untold time and resources in an attempt to stave off extinction for the condor. How this will play out in the end no one yet knows.

To best avoid crowds at Lake Powell, paddle there in the off-season. If possible, avoid weekends even during the off-season.

Trip Description

Launch your boat at the main ramp at Halls Crossing. There are several parking lots in the vicinity of the launch ramp. Paddle north out of the launching and moorage area until you can see due east, which is up-lake. Then paddle east along the south shore. Within 1 mile you will pass the small cove where the car-ferry landing is located. A double-pronged inlet, 0.7 mile farther along, runs 1 mile south from the shore at full pool.

There are two 0.25-mile deep inlets in the south shore 0.7 mile farther. Beyond them to the east, you can easily see the first of many vertical cliffs that make up a stretch of shoreline in the main lake. Paddle to the east end of these cliffs, which mark the entrance to Moki Canyon (4 miles from launch). Moki is a major canyon and worth exploring if you have the time (because Forgotten Canyon—your destination—is 7 miles up-lake from Moki).

Moki Canyon side trip:

Paddle slightly south of east, into Moki Canyon. The Park Service has placed a buoy at the entrance of major canyons, and the one you pass here indicates appropriately moki canyon. At 0.5 mile into the canyon, a branch inlet leads northeast for 0.7 mile. The stone walls of this inlet, like others in the canyon, are spectacular, but there are no unusual features in this branch. Back in the main Moki Canyon, look for ruins and petroglyphs on the north bank a few hundred yards east of the branch inlet. Continue up-canyon 1 mile, to where another branch inlet leads southeast for 0.5 mile. This is an interesting branch with vertical walls and an echo-chamber alcove at the end, which lies 90° to the axis of the inlet. Back in the main Moki Canyon, paddle east 0.7 mile, past two northeast-trending inlets on the north bank. The first one is 0.5 mile long, while the second is shorter but has a neat cave at the water line into which you can paddle your boat. Continue east 0.8 mile up Moki Canyon from the inlets to a fork in the canyon (3 miles from canyon mouth). North Gulch is the left branch, con-tinuing east for another mile. Approximately 0.2 mile beyond full-pool level are ruins in the cliffs on the north side of North Gulch. Moki Canyon continues in an easterly direction for another 1.5 miles. There are two ruins above the water on the north side, and another ruin about 0.3 mile upstream, beyond the lake.

Continue east up-lake, past the Moki Canyon entrance. Here the main lake makes a lazy 180° bend left and, if you like, you can cut the corner, coming close to the inside point. Just west of the point along the north shore, the water is very shallow and the shoreline gentle. Buoys are placed here to mark the extent of the deeper water. There are slickrock islands where you can land, small inlets, and some sand beaches. Alas, there is no real shade here, only a few scrub willows scattered about. Still, it is a good place for a swim.

Continue north around the point, then cut across the channel again, if the water is calm, to the next point, which is 2 miles northwest. Along the way, you may pass red buoys "102" or "102A," which mark the shallows you will paddle over as you round this next point (6 miles from launch). Once around this point, you can see 6 miles up-lake in a north-northeasterly direction. Paddle up-lake along the east shore. This segment has abrupt banks, a few shallow, curved inlets, and longer-distance views. Hansen Creek Canyon leads northwest from the main channel 2.5 miles north of the last point you rounded (8.5 miles from launch). This 4-mile-long canyon has gently sloping banks, which indicate that the water is shallow along shore. While campsites can be easily found, there are no remarkable features in this inlet. On the east shore, 0.5 mile beyond the mouth of Hansen Creek Canyon, Crystal Springs Canyon leads southeast for 2 miles. This narrow inlet—like many others—is beautiful, impressive in its steep walls and fluted shoreline. There are no vis-ible ruins within this canyon.

Paddle northeast 1.7 miles from the mouth of Crystal Springs Canyon to the mouth of Forgotten Canyon. (Midpoint in this segment, two inlet spurs lead eastward nearly 0.5 mile from the main channel.) Turn right (east) into Forgotten Canyon at the buoy identifying it (10.7 miles from launch). The Park Service maintains a floating restroom and pump-out station just inside the canyon mouth. Head east, and in 0.7 mile an inlet leads south 0.5 mile. Continue east 0.2 mile in Forgotten Canyon to where a narrow inlet leads east 1 mile. Pass this inlet also and—still in the main channel—paddle east approximately 0.7 mile.

Keep a lookout in the alcoves along the north shore until you spot Defiance House, a restored ruin (1.6 miles from the canyon mouth). Against the red-rock wall, the structures—made of the same red rock—do not stand out. However, the greater-than-life-size figures of three warriors painted in a light ochre color *do* contrast. These pictographs convey a sense of purposeful defense to the observer, hence the name "Defiance House." The Park Service has *hardened* the ruins by replacing mud mortar with cement mortar of the same color, and making the ruin stable enough to withstand visitors. There is an above-ground dwelling, an underground kiva, and several kitchen pits.

There are sand beaches and camping possibilities on both shore—from Defiance House east to the end of the inlet about 0.5 mile farther. When the inlet shallows to a creek, there are possible campsites on either shore, which cannot be reached by houseboats. To return to Halls Crossing, paddle the above route in reverse.

Alternate or Additional Trips

(The author has paddled all canyons and inlets from Forgotten Canyon west and north to the center of the Escalante Arm; suggestions about other trips are from charts, maps, and research.) Even a glance at a map of Lake Powell will tell you there are *many* different trips or combinations of trips that you can paddle here. Having enough space is not a problem. The issues are those of paddling on lake segments small enough or protected enough to remove the stress factors for beginners, and to avoid powerboat traffic. Wahweap Marina near Glen Canyon Dam is by far the largest facility on the lake. And the broad bays in the western 30 miles of Lake Powell are big water, with lots of powerboat traffic. For this reason, the paddler may find a trip on Powell more enjoyable if the western end of the lake is avoided. So, what is possible on the remaining portions of the lake?

As a destination Rainbow Bridge involves about 50 miles of paddling (one way) from either Bullfrog, Halls Crossing, or Wahweap. This mileage does not allow for exploring the canyons along the way. Rainbow Bridge is a National Monument within the National Recreation Area. No camping is allowed within the monument, which is a favorite destination for tourist excursion boats. Still, the huge natural bridge is a worthy destination and, when the long paddle there is interrupted by exploration into side canyons, the trip nearly achieves expedition status. There are enough arches, caves, and other geological and archaeological features along the way to keep a paddler interested for many days.

The Escalante Arm, a major north-trending canyon with its own interesting side canyons, offers arches, caves, and ruins adjoining one of the newest wilderness areas in the country. The Escalante Arm is about 28 paddling miles west of Halls Crossing.

The upper lake, between Hite and Halls Crossing, is about 50 miles of narrowing main channel with some wider bays. There are not as many side

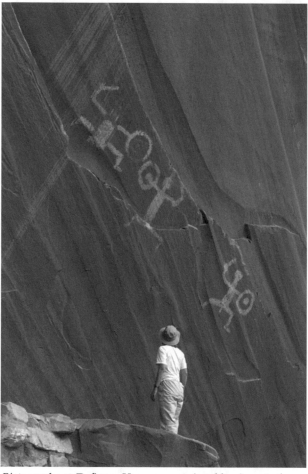

Pictographs at Defiance House were painted by Ancestral Puebloans between A.D. 1000-1100

canyons along this segment, which might be suitable for a one-way passage if a transportation shuttle can be arranged.

The San Juan Arm, which joins the main lake about 8 miles west of the Escalante Arm, is approximately 40 miles of channel and minor side canyons, with no services of any kind along the way or at the end. Some 4WD roads reach the lake here from the Navajo Indian Reservation to the south. There are a few, scattered petroglyph sites, but no ruins adjacent to the water. Powerboat traffic is light in this section.

Contacts
National Park Service
Glen Canyon National Recreation Area
PO Box 1507
Page, AZ 86040
(520) 608-6404

Across lake from Halls Crossing:
National Park Service
Bullfrog Visitor Center
(435) 684-7400

Halls Crossing Campground
(435) 684-7000

Paddling into the shade was a welcome relief. But more than shade, the stone of the huge alcove towering above the water seemed to have a cooling effect. We maneuvered the boat deeper into the alcove, almost touching the desert-varnish tapestry that streaked the towering red wall. Above us, the wall sloped up and outward, sharp against the light blue, heat-shimmering sky.

Then we saw the line in the sandstone 15 feet above, where moisture seeped down a few inches from a horizontal crack on the cliff surface. The yards-long hanging garden featured a bush, precariously anchored in the sandstone, and a brilliant green line of maidenhair ferns. At the other end, a single, thriving columbine sent out a half-dozen flowers. Out of nowhere as we watched, a hummingbird zoomed in, sampled a flower and, as fast as it had appeared, disappeared around the alcove edge.

Reluctantly we left the alcove and paddled up-canyon, keeping as much as possible in the shade cast by vertical walls. The afternoon wore on, giving little sign that the 90° air would cool off refreshingly as the sun dropped. Then we reached a south-facing alcove, where two powerboats were moored to the talus slope below the overhang. At first we couldn't spot the ruins themselves, but there was no mistaking the pictographs. There, on the smooth sandstone of the alcove, three warriors stood men-

acingly with weapons raised and round shields poised. The light ochre pictographs practically shouted Here! This is the place!

As we stroked slowly ashore, one of the moored boats left—with the engine on low idle—slower than the 5 mph limit, as if in respect for this site. We moored our double kayak, and climbed up the trail as the other party was leaving. When we reached the ruin, we were alone. The residence, with smoke-stained, wooden-pole ceiling, was made of sandstone that had fallen from the alcove walls. Adjacent, reached by a wooden ladder that disappeared into a dark hole in the ground, was a single kiva. Several, walled kitchen pits nearby completed what remained of the complex.

About such a ruin is a feeling that is difficult to describe. A presence lingers, and you find yourself talking in soft, hushed tones. The design and construction skills of the ancient ones are right there in front of you. When did they leave? Why? How many people lived here? What is the meaning of the warrior pictograph? How did they paint it so high off the ground? Noticeable, too, is that vast expanse of smooth, red wall at ground level, against which the structures nestle, extending many yards on either side. No graffiti. No mark other than the pictograph. With what veneration did these people approach their environment? Was graffiti taboo? Were children disciplined?

That familiar feeling of reverence came over me as we left the ruins, as it always does when I visit some site or activity rooted in antiquity. Then we were in the kayak, paddling slowly away, the gurgle of our sharp turn reverberating in the alcove.

The moon was up before we completed evening camp chores. A short distance away the alcove cliff loomed dark, as if unimpressed with the sparkle of moonlight on the water riffles. The canyon was silent. If we hadn't just visited that afternoon, we wouldn't know that the ruin was there. Then we were in the tent, slipping into dreams after the long day's paddle. Are those voices from the past I hear? Most likely they are only some animal in the night. But it is hard to be certain.

Appendix 1—Map and Boating-Regulation Resources

For Maps

USGS Topographical maps, indexes, and symbol explanations may be purchased from:

Western Distribution Branch
U.S. Geological Survey
PO Box 25286
Denver Federal Center
Denver, CO 80225
(303) 202-4700
The Geological Survey now accepts credit cards, which greatly facilitates ordering.

For same-day shipping of topographical maps (although at a higher cost from these non-government sources):

Powers Elevation Co.
(303) 321-2217
Located in Colorado, this company can supply any USGS map.

Map Centre, Inc.
2611 University Ave.
San Diego, CA 92104-3830
(619) 291-3830
USGS topos, NOAA charts, other maps (credit card orders)

The Map Center
2440 Bancroft Way
Berkeley, CA 94704
(510) 841-6277, 841-0858 (Fax)
USGS topos, NOAA charts, other maps (credit card orders)

For Boating Regulations

Boaters' Handbooks or brochures summarizing state boating laws are available from:

State of California

California Resources Agency
Department of Boating & Waterways
2000 Evergreen St. #100
Sacramento, CA 95815-3888
(916) 263-4326

State of Arizona

Arizona Game & Fish Department
2221 West Greenway Rd.
Phoenix, AZ 85023
(602) 942-3000

State of Oregon

Oregon Marine Board
PO Box 14145
Salem, OR 97309-5065
(503) 378-8587

State of Utah

Utah State Parks & Recreation
1594 West N. Temple #116
Salt Lake City, UT 84116
(801) 538-7220

State of Washington

Washington State Parks & Recreation Commission
Boating Safety Division
7150 Cleanwater Ln.
Olympia, WA 98504-2650
(360) 902-8500

Appendix 2—Recommended Reading

Geology

Alt, David D., and Donald W. Hyndman, *Roadside Geology of Oregon, Roadside Geology Series*, Mountain Press Publishing Company, 1991.

Alt, David D., and Donald W. Hyndman, *Roadside Geology of Northern and Central California*, Roadside Geology Series, Mountain Press Publishing Company, 2000.

Alt, David D., and Donald W. Hyndman, *Roadside Geology of Washington, Roadside Geology Series*, Mountain Press Publishing Company, 1986.

Chronic, Halka, *Roadside Geology of Utah, Roadside Geology Series*, Mountain Press Publishing Company, 1988.

Chronic, Halka, *Roadside Geology of Arizona, Roadside Geology Series*, Mountain Press Publishing Company, 1986.

Price, L. Greer, *Grand Canyon Geology*, Grand Canyon Association, Grand Canyon, Arizona, 1999.

Flora & Fauna

Spellenberg, Richard, *The Audubon Society Field Guide to North American Wildflowers,*Western Region, Alfred A. Knopf, 1979.

Udvardy, Miklos D.F., and John Farrand, Jr., *The Audubon Society Field Guide to North American Birds, Western Region*, Alfred A. Knopf, rev. 1997.

Whitaker, John O., Jr., *The Audubon Society Field Guide to North American Mammals*, Alfred A. Knopf, 1988.

Kayaking

Burch, David, *Fundamentals of Kayak Navigation*, Globe Pequot Press, 1987.

Hutchinson, Derek C., *Derek C. Hutchinson's Guide to Expedition Kayaking on Sea & Open Water*, The Globe Pequot Press, 1990.

Hutchinson, Derek C., *The Complete Book of Sea Kayaking*, The Globe Pequot Press, 1994.

Keating, W.R., *Survival in Cold Water*, Blackwell Scientific Publishers, 1969.

First Aid for the Outdoors

Darvill, Fred T., Jr., M.D., *Mountaineering Medicine*, 14th ed., Wilderness Press, 1998.

Forgey, William W., *Wilderness Medicine*, ICS Books, 1987.

Wilkerson, James A., M.D., *Medicine for Mountaineering*, The Mountaineers Books, 1985.

Kayaking on open water entails unavoidable risk that every kayaker assumes and must be aware of and respect. The fact that a trip is described in this book is not a representation that it will be safe for you. Kayaking trips vary greatly in difficulty and in the degree of conditioning and skill one needs to enjoy them safely. On some trips the area may have changed or conditions may have deteriorated since the descriptions were written. Trip conditions change even from day to day, owing to weather and other factors. A trip that is safe on a calm day or for a highly conditioned, experienced, properly equipped kayaker may be completely unsafe for someone else or unsafe under adverse weather conditions.

You can minimize your risks on the water by being knowledgeable, prepared and alert. There is not space in this book for a general treatise on safety on the water, but there are a number of good books and instruction courses on the subject and you should take advantage of them to increase your knowledge. Just as important, you should always be aware of your own limitations and of conditions existing when and where you are kayaking. If conditions are dangerous, or if you're not prepared to deal with them safely, choose a different trip, or don't go at all. It's better to have wasted a drive than to be the subject of a rescue. These warnings are not intended to scare you off the water. However, one element of the beauty, freedom and excitement of kayaking is the presence of risks that do not confront us at home. When you kayak you assume those risks. They can be met safely, but only if you exercise your own independent judgement and common sense. The author and the publisher of this book disclaim any liability or loss resulting from the use of this book.

Index

Page numbers for maps and photographs are in *italic*.